I was that man on the couch, and at my largest I weighed 455 pounds. When I finally got moving and lost more than 200 pounds, it transformed me on the outside and, even more, so on the inside. *Get Off the Couch* will give you a clear plan of action that will work for you. Steve shows you how to change your life both physically and spiritually.

Ken Andrews
Co-founder, RetroFit Ministries
Contestant, *The Biggest Loser* (Season 11)

If you struggle with your weight or have health-related issues, or know someone who does, this is the book for you! Pastor Steve has written a uniquely practical and scripturally sound tool to help you take care of the body God has given you. As a man who has walked the talk, Steve has packed this book with lots of encouragement and great manly advice to win the battle.

Dave Brown
Chairman, Foundation for Manhood
Director, Washington Area Coalition of Men's Ministries

The dictionary defines "movement" as "an act of changing physical location or position or *of having this changed*." I placed the emphasis on the last part because if you don't get off the couch and get moving, you could end up with the coroner "moving" you! We need each other, and Steve does an excellent job of providing a plan that will help you get moving *on your own* and become a healthier you!

Scott Davis
Comedian and Author, *If My Body Is a Temple, Then I Was a Megachurch*

Steve Reynolds has been an inspiration in the pulpit for many years as he has shared the truth of the gospel. Now, Steve is an inspiration at the refrigerator and the couch as he guides us in maintaining healthy lifestyles. There is no question that one of the most difficult things to do is eat healthy and exercise. Steve, through his own life experience, gives us great wisdom as to how we can make this a priority . . . and a reality in our own lives. Read this book—your health depends on it.

Jonathan Falwell
Pastor, Thomas Road Baptist Church

If I knew nothing else about *Get Off the Couch* than the fact it was written by a Bible-based pastor, I would read it. Barring any medical reasons, you gaining weight is a spiritual battle, and food may be your idol. What better fitness trainer than a pastor who knows how to apply God's Word to your health. Steve Reynolds is a modern-day apostle Paul—armed and dangerous!

Ihab John Ibrahim
Medical Doctor

Steve Reynolds has a passion for men to lose weight, get fit and be all they can be. Women will flock to buy this book for the man they love, and men are going to appreciate Steve's no-nonsense approach to health and total wellness.

Carole Lewis
National Director, First Place 4 Health
Author, *Live Life Right Here, Right Now*

I've known Steve since the 1970s, when we were football teammates at Liberty University. As a running back, I depended on Steve to open big holes for me—and he was big enough to open gaping holes! Over the years, I've had the privilege of training more than 1,300 NFL players and some of the greatest athletes in the NBA, MLB, MLS, NHL, PGA and in professional tennis, and I stress to my pros that total fitness means being physically, mentally and spiritually fit. No matter what your current level of fitness, *Get Off the Couch* will motivate you to get up and move! We all need to be the most fit Kingdom players possible.

Chip Smith
Author, *Football Training Like the Pros*

I believe you must be able to lead yourself before you can properly lead others. One area of importance is physical fitness. If you do not get adequate exercise, eat the right fuel, and get enough sleep, you limit your effectiveness. *Get Off the Couch* shows how to experience personal renewal and maximize your energy. Steve Reynolds lays out a clear plan for getting the most out of your body and making the greatest impact for God.

Steve Stroope
Lead Pastor, Lake Pointe Church
Author, *Tribal Church*

Being an NFL agent, most people think I spend a lot of time on the couch watching sports. It is true I love sports and closely follow it, but I still make time for regular exercise. *Get Off the Couch* is my kind of book, and I highly recommend it. It shows men how to spend time in their man cave watching some sports and still take care of their health. So, let's get off the couch!

Robert B. Walker
President and CEO, Unlimited Success Sports Management, Inc.

Steve Reynolds

The "Anti-Fat Pastor" and Bestselling Author of *Bod4God* | with M. G. Ellis

GET OFF THE
COUCH

A Man's **A.C.T.I.O.N.** Plan

6 MOTIVATORS TO HELP YOU
LOSE WEIGHT AND *START LIVING*

Regal

For more information and
special offers from Regal Books, email us at
subscribe@regalbooks.com

Published by Regal
From Gospel Light
Ventura, California, U.S.A.
www.regalbooks.com
Printed in the U.S.A.

Note: The information contained in this book is intended to be solely for informational
and educational purposes. Please consult a medical or health professional before beginning
this or any other weight-loss or physical fitness program.

Library of Congress Cataloging-in-Publication Data
Reynolds, Steve, Pastor.
Get off the couch / Steve Reynolds.
p. cm.
Includes bibliographical references.
ISBN 978-0-8307-6516-4
1. Men—Health and hygiene. 2. Health—Psychological aspects.
3. Mind and body. I. Title.
RA777.8.R49 2012
613'.04234—dc23
2012027507

Rights for publishing this book outside the U.S.A. or in non-English languages are
administered by Gospel Light Worldwide, an international not-for-profit ministry.
For additional information, please visit www.glww.org, email info@glww.org, or write to
Gospel Light Worldwide, 1957 Eastman Avenue, Ventura, CA 93003, U.S.A.

To order copies of this book and other Regal products in bulk quantities,
please contact us at 1-800-446-7735.

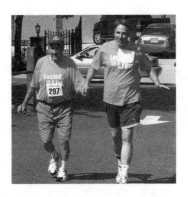

This book is dedicated to my dad, Alfred Dean Reynolds.

I love this picture of you and me completing the
Losing to Live 5K run together. At 81 years old, you are still living a full
and active life, including walking every day. You are an inspiration to me
and to our family. Thank you for making God the center of our home and
for passing on to our family the godly values that were instilled in you by
your parents. I love you, Dad.

He who has knowledge spares his words,
and a man of understanding is of a calm spirit.

PROVERBS 17:27

Contents

Acknowledgments

This was a TEAM project. I greatly appreciate the group of people who helped me develop this book, including:

My family, for always supporting me. I love you all very much.

My church family, members and staff of Capital Baptist Church in Annandale, Virginia, for your loyal support. It is truly an honor to serve as your pastor.

My friends Gary, Jana, Jaden and Josalyn Moritz, for your major contribution in creating this book. It would have never happened without your help. I love you all very much.

My writing assistant, Gwen Ellis, for your contributions to the book.

My friend Randy Miller, Graduate Research Assistance Librarian at Liberty University in Lynchburg, Virginia, for providing valuable research for this book.

My photographer, Randy Ritter, who took most of the pictures in this book.

My men's focus group, who reviewed this book and provided valuable input.

My Reflection and Discussion Question team, who helped create and shape that section of the book.

My group of men who contributed testimonies and were willing to be transparent and share their journey.

My partners in the Losing to Live weight-loss program, who are with me on the front lines of the fight against obesity.

My publisher, Regal Books, and especially Bill Greig III, Stan Jantz, Kim Bangs and Mark Weising, for your guidance in producing a quality book.

My readers—you honor me for taking time out of your busy lives to read this book.

Be the Man God Created You to Be!

by Nelson Searcy

I can relate to the journey that led Steve to creating the *Get off the Couch* A.C.T.I.O.N. plan. A few years ago, I ranked among the millions of men in America who desperately need to dropkick the sedentary lifestyle and get moving toward a healthier life. As a church leader, I had spent my entire career building God's kingdom, but I had let His temple—my body—fall into disrepair. My physical health just wasn't of much concern to me, even though I had read Paul's words in 1 Corinthians 6:19-20 many times:

> Do you not know that your body is the temple of the Holy Spirit who is in you, whom you have from God, and you are not your own? For you were bought at a price; therefore glorify God in your body and in your spirit, which are God's.

Like most people, I connected these verses with sexual sin—and sexual sin only—though they have a much wider implication. Through some in-depth study and lots of prayer, I began to take hold of the weighty reality that my body was the living, breathing and walking-around temple of God's Spirit. So is yours. Our bodies are the dwelling place of the Alpha and Omega. Our skin, bones and fleshy guts are home to the Most High. That's a humbling thought, isn't it?

As they say, the truth will set you free. Thanks to my new perspective on God's plan for my body, I began to shift my entire mindset toward physical health. I started thinking, *If God has entrusted me with this earthly vessel—*

Before**After**

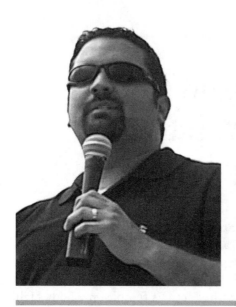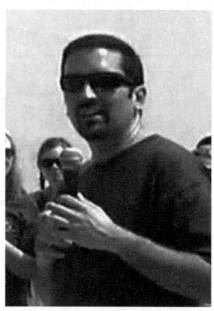

not to mention all the work and plans He has for me while living in it—where do I get off trashing it by eating what I want and letting it atrophy? Where do you? How can we stomach treating ourselves so poorly that we can't fully engage in God's purposes for us?

Of course, we come up with a lot of excuses to defend against these types of questions. We've been conditioned to think we have a family history of hearty eaters and big bellies, or we're just "big-boned," or we don't have time to exercise. On and on it goes as we build our case. All of these excuses—and the hundreds of others we create in a desperate attempt to stay within our carefully constructed comfort zone—keep us from embracing the truth that God wants us to live full and active lives and accomplish the things He put us here to do. We have a responsibility in cooperating with Him to make that happen.

In Steve's first book *Bod4God* (which I also highly recommend), he breaks down many of our health excuses by detailing exactly what the Bible has to say about how we should treat our bodies and what we should eat to keep them effectively fueled. With *Get off the Couch*, Steve tackles the other half of the equation we all wrestle with when it comes to getting ourselves healthy: intentionally getting up and moving our bodies in a way that will keep us strong for the long haul. As Steve points out, life is too short and too precious to waste, and God has invested way too much in us for us to sit around squandering our potential and allowing things like poor food choices and lack of exercise to hold us back from all He has in store. In the pages ahead, he will challenge you to *man up* and dive into simple changes that can transform your health.

Getting off the couch, for me, meant making a decision to take control of my health and putting an exercise plan behind that decision. I committed to changing myself from being someone who didn't even like to walk very far to becoming someone who could be considered a habitual runner. If you had told me five or six years ago that I would start running several times per week and actually enjoy it, I would have called you crazy. But the day came when I knew I had to man up and make a change.

A friend recommended an MP3 running program called *Couch to 5K*. As the title implies, the program takes a person who is used to almost no physical activity and guides him through an incremental process that results in being able to run for 30 minutes without stopping. The first day I laced up my sneakers and cued up my iPod to give the program a try, I had a hard time running for 60 seconds straight. I remember stumbling back into my New York City apartment—after much more walking than running—and saying to my wife, "I don't know if I can do this. Maybe it's not for me."

But after a day's rest, I tried it again. And then again. And then one more time. Slowly but surely, my endurance began to build. After about eight weeks, I was running for the full 30 minutes. Running has now become an important part of my life, and I miss it when I don't get it in. I'm not saying I'm always eager to jump into my running shoes; sometimes I still have to force myself out the door. But even on those days, I always finish my run with a great sense of satisfaction that I am doing my part to keep this body that God gave me in prime working condition.

I tell you my story to say this: If I can get up off of the couch and get the upper hand on my weight and health issues, so can you. If the men whose stories you'll read about in these pages can do it, so can you. You have what it takes to get from where you are to where you want to be. Decide to honor God with your entire being, including the body he has given you, and dive headlong into the A.C.T.I.O.N. plan Steve outlines.

Steve is not a theorist—the plan he proposes in *Get off the Couch* comes as a direct result of his own personal experience and success. As you'll see, there came a point in Steve's life when he had to man up, and there will come a point when you will have to man up as well. Speaking from the other side of the (ongoing) journey, I can tell you that taking the necessary action to get your physical health under control is more than worth the effort. There's no better gift you can give yourself or those who love you.

This is your life. It's time to be the man God created you to be. I will be praying for you along the way!

Nelson Searcy
Founder and Lead Pastor, The Journey Church in New York City
    and Boca Raton, Florida
Author, *The Greatness Principle* and *The Generosity Ladder*

In Sickness and in Health
by Debbie Reynolds

When Steve Reynolds, my 340-pound husband, came through the door after visiting his doctor, I knew something was up.

"What did the doctor say, Steve?" I asked while holding my breath.

"He said I have diabetes."

I stared at him a long moment. "Diabetes?" I whispered.

"That's what he said. 'Type 2 diabetes.'"

"What are you going to do? What did the doctor say would help?"

"Well, he said I'm too heavy—'obese,' he called me. He said if I lose weight and begin exercising, I have a chance to beat this."

I exhaled. "Then that's what you have to do."

"Nah. I told him to just give me some pills."

"And did he?"

Steve nodded.

"I wish you'd try exercise and eat better. I know I feel better when I do, and you will too."

"I'm just going to take the pills."

I can tell you, I was scared. We were only in our forties, and our children were still young and in our home. I did not want to be a widow with three kids to care for. A little research confirmed my worst fears. Steve's condition was life-threatening. Becoming a widow was a real possibility.

It was hard to believe how far we had come from our wedding day, when the two of us had stood at the altar in the best shape of our lives. We were so young and in love and full of life. We said those words in our wedding vows, "In sickness and in health"—but who really imagines the "in sickness" part when you are looking and feeling your best on one of the

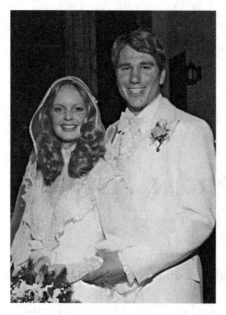

happiest days of your life? I even remember us saying whenever we saw an older, overweight couple, "We will never look like that." We went so far as to promise each other that we would never let ourselves go and gain a lot of weight. But here we were, living the "in sickness" part of our wedding vows, and it terrified me. The problem was that, like so many people, we had a goal to be healthy but no action plan to make that goal happen.

If Steve was scared, he didn't let on. He was determined to just take the pills and avoid eating right and exercising. Nothing I said or did changed his mind. What could I do?

I didn't know if Steve would ever change. I knew that while I might want to nag him about the issue, it wouldn't work. So I decided I would be loving and supportive of him. I would pray that God would put a desire in his heart to get serious about his condition. In the meantime, I could provide an environment that would help promote change. I could cook more healthy foods. I could become more active in order to set a good example. I could invite Steve to go for a walk with me. I could plan activities that were fun and that would keep not only Steve and I active but the kids as well. I thought back to the kinds of things Steve enjoyed doing when he was younger, and we did some of those activities together—like playing golf.

Steve began to think about his condition, and after a while he began to wonder if he *could* beat diabetes. I held my breath and waited. He decided he might as well give the doctor's advice a try. He had nothing to lose but weight. What I didn't know then was that his pursuit of health was going to become bigger than just caring for his body. His ideas about health were going to spread nationwide and impact many people. He would become known as the "Anti-Fat Pastor." I was thrilled with the changes he was making, and I determined to do everything I could to help him succeed.

Soon, Steve's decision to change affected every member of our family—even his mother. A thorough cupboard cleaning helped us lose the unhealthy treats. Gone were the chips and dips. Gone were the cookies, cakes and other pastries. And, most of all, gone was the ice cream. Steve could eat astonishing amounts of ice cream. A nightly bowl of ice cream was not a dessert; it was a tradition—a necessary part of life—a fitting end to a day.

Steve has always done the grocery shopping at our house. Now, he began to buy healthy snacks of fruit, low-fat cheese and whole-grain crackers. When someone wanted a snack, healthy food was all that was available. Where we had hardly ever thought to have a glass of water, we now made drinking it a big part of our life.

Steve soon began to lose weight, and the church members asked him how he was doing it. He told them about the small changes he was making and how they were helping him to drop the weight and feel better. Bod4God was born in Steve's mind. The church began having 12-week "Losing to Live" competitions, which teach people how to eat, why exercise is important, why God wants us to live in healthy bodies, and how making small changes can have a huge impact on our health.

Life changed for our family, and I am so glad. We used to go on vacation and pretty much just sit around and eat. Last year, we took a vacation to the west coast of Costa Rica. It was the most active vacation we've ever had. We went zip-lining, rode four-wheelers on the beach, and went to a park where there is an active volcano. We hiked a steep hill and climbed up on some of the volcanic rock so we could look down into a lake fed by warm waters from the volcano. We managed the uphill hike just fine. We had such a wonderful time that every member of the family can't wait to go back.

There is another part of healthy living that I want to talk about, and that is getting your man to the doctor for regular checkups. Men in their forties need to have screenings for diabetes, high-cholesterol, high blood pressure and prostate cancer, followed by yearly checkups. These are all silent killers that a man might not know he has until it is too late. A high percentage of men have prostate cancer by the time they are 80, and for some it starts much earlier. If the man in your life won't make an appointment with the doctor, do it for him and tell him why: you don't want anything to happen to him; you need him; you want to keep him around. For some men, setting an annual appointment near a birthday is a good reminder that a year has gone by. (In fact, one of the annual cancer-walk events has a slogan, "We're all about birthdays.") One of the best gifts any of us can have is another birthday. So get your man to the doctor, and do your part to keep him alive and healthy.

Life is much different now than it was that day when Steve looked at me and told me he was sick. The best part is that he now no longer has diabetes, high blood pressure or high cholesterol. He has so much energy that most people can't keep up with him. He puts in long days at our church, and now he travels to tell others that they can also have a Bod4God. He has found a calling and a passion for helping people of all kinds and ages find health. God is using him to change people's lives here on earth and for eternity. I am very proud of him. I am proud of his sticking to the plan and dropping well over a hundred pounds. I am proud of his concern for others, and I am his first and best cheerleader. And I am so grateful to God for giving us these precious years together. We are blessed people.

Pastor Steve Before

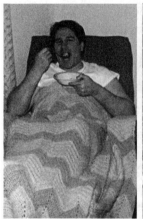 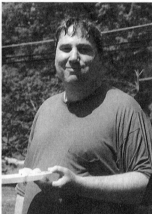 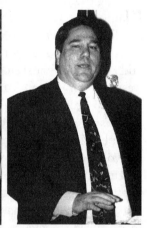

Pastor Steve After

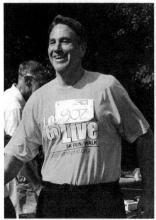 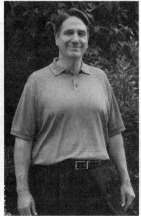 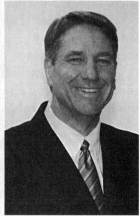

A Man's A.C.T.I.O.N. Plan

Action! Every guy loves action and adventure. Action movies . . . fast car chases . . . war . . . sports . . . anything that will get our adrenaline pumping. We live for danger, risk and fun. As little boys, we dreamed of being super heroes, warriors, sports stars, fireman and police officers rushing into perilous situations to save the day. We were always looking for the next adventure.

Well, you are about to embark on a brand new one—an exciting journey. This adventure is your life. You may not feel like much of a conqueror these days. Your current physical condition may have you feeling defeated and lost. But things are about change. In this book, you are about to explore six actions that will make you victorious and keep you from being a victim. These six actions, found in the following A.C.T.I.O.N. acrostic, will enable you to launch your new adventure:

Aware:	Be *aware* of the seriousness of your physical condition and understand that your body matters to God.
Commit:	*Commit* to living a disciplined life and to winning over temptation.
Transform:	*Transform* the way you think and the way you live.
Incorporate:	*Incorporate* healthy eating habits and exercise into your daily life.
Organize:	*Organize* a team of people to help you win.
Navigate:	Create an A.C.T.I.O.N. plan for healthy living so you can *navigate* your way to leaving a lasting legacy.

The Parts of the Plan

The six sections in *Get Off the Couch* focus on each of these six action steps that you need to incorporate in your life in order to get off the couch and into shape. Each section/action has two chapters dedicated to introducing and explaining the principles you need to start applying to your life in order to win in the area of your health. Within each chapter, you will find the following:

- A *key Bible verse* at the beginning of each chapter to meditate on that will aid and reinforce the action step (these are listed in appendix E).

- A *story* from a guy just like you who has gotten off the couch and started to take action to change his life.

- A *Man Up* section that contains: (1) an *Eat Up* section that will give you great eating tips and suggestions, and (2) a *Pump Up* section that will give you suggestions for exercises you can use to get into shape.

- A *Check Up sidebar* that will inform you on the risks of obesity and the benefits of getting healthy.[1]

- *Reflection and discussion questions,* which are designed to help you dig deeper into the principles and practices introduced within the chapter.

- *My Personal Game Plan for Getting in Shape,* which you can use to start tracking what specific steps you are going to take in implementing the actions from the chapter.

Each of these sections is vitally important and crucial in determining whether or not you will succeed in producing life change. I have also included a Progress Report in appendix A of this book that you can use to keep track of your progress through this journey, in addition to some other useful tools that will help you.

The Participants in the Plan

This book was designed so that you could read it alone or use it as a study within a small-group setting. For some of you, reading *Get Off the Couch* will be something you do alone—a personal journey as you reflect on your health and wellness. However, you might also want to consider reading and discussing this book as part of a men's small-group, with a Losing to Live weight loss competition, or just by asking a good buddy to do it along with you.

Another good option is to discuss the material in this book as part of a First Place 4 Health group. This ministry has played a major part in my weight-loss journey, and it is a vital part of the wellness ministry of the church I pastor. Founded in 1981, First Place 4 Health is a Christian weight-loss and healthy living program that has had groups in more than 12,000 churches across the country. Unlike other health and fitness programs, First Place 4 Health emphasizes a biblical approach to weight loss and focuses on improving every area of a person's life—mentally, emotionally, physically and spiritually. Members meet at scheduled times to encourage and support one another, share struggles and triumphs, and study the Word of God. First Place 4 Health offers a series of Bible studies, which address many issues of everyday life and provide members with opportunities to grow together in Christ.

The Process for the Plan

I want to encourage you to take your time as you go through this book. While you are reading, you are going to be learning how to let go of a lot of bad habits, how to start producing change, and how to form healthier habits. That is going to take time. *I suggest that you go through a chapter a week and not only read it, but also start putting the principles discussed in that chapter into practice.* Twelve weeks is not a long time compared to the rest of your life. This is your time—your time to change, your time to start living again.

This Book Is for You

Congratulations! It was a risky move just picking up this book and beginning to read it. Now, I want you to take another step and keep reading. I am going to walk with you on this journey as I share my heart with you, man to man. I will share some things that will make you laugh, some things that will make you think, and some things that will change how you view yourself. I will challenge you to keep moving. I am also going to say to you, "Man Up! It's time to change!" Yes, this book is about action, but it is also about your re-action. So stay focused. Let me help you be the man you want to be. Let me share my story with you and explain how I went from being a conqueror on the football field to a lazy bum in a La-Z-Boy, and then how I got off the couch and back into shape. We'll get started by talking about the first action step!

Pastor Steve Reynolds

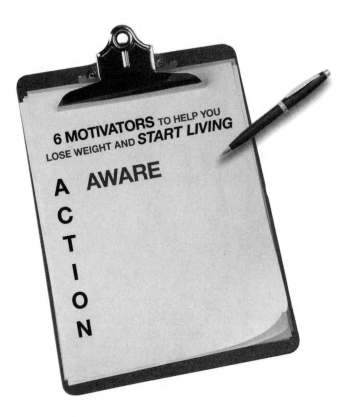

Aware

The journey toward a healthier life begins by becoming *aware* of the seriousness of your physical condition and the fact that your body matters to God. What do you know about your body? Do you know your current cholesterol level, your blood pressure, your blood sugar levels, your body mass index (BMI) or even what you currently weigh? Are you *aware* of the fact that God carefully crafted your body and that He loves you and wants you to be in good health? It's time to face the facts regarding your health, and it's time to start living a life that reflects the image of the One who created you.

Chapter 1

Get in the Game

I can do all things through Christ who strengthens me.
PHILIPPIANS 4:13

Football! What guy doesn't get pumped up by that word? Some years ago, there was a movie called *Rudy*. In the story, Rudy wants to play football for Notre Dame more than almost anything else in life. There are a couple of problems, though. His grades are lousy, he doesn't have the money for any college, and even though his heart for the game is huge, he is only about five feet tall and weighs a little more than 100 pounds.

After Rudy's best friend dies, he realizes that life is short and that if he is going to do what he wants to do, he has to get off the bench and engage life. So he ignores the obstacles in his path and heads for Notre Dame. Once there, he is at a loss as to how to reach his dream. He can't even get into the college.

Rudy meets a graduate student at Notre Dame who helps him improve his grades. He is accepted into Holy Cross Junior College in South Bend and begins spending his time studying and working as a groundskeeper at Notre Dame's Knute Rockne Stadium. Rudy learns that he is dyslexic, and Holy Cross puts a plan in place to help him learn in spite of the disability. His grades improve, and after three semesters he is finally granted acceptance into Notre Dame. There is, however, no acceptance to the football team.

The courageous and never-say-die Rudy soon convinces the coach to give him a spot on the practice squad. Rudy's determination and passion for the game are legendary, yet the coach still overlooks him when it comes time to suit up for a game, even though all the other seniors are doing so. This doesn't fly with the other seniors on the team, and one by one they walk into the coach's office and lay their jerseys on his desk. They demand that the coach allows Rudy to suit up in their places. The coach, realizing his back is against the wall, gives in and lets Rudy suit up for the final home game against Georgia Tech.

The team captain, Steele, gives Rudy the honor of leading the team out of the tunnel onto the playing field, but then Rudy sits on the bench. Notre Dame leads when the coach sends all the seniors to the field—all, that is, except Rudy. Steele and the assistant coaches protest. The Notre Dame bench starts a "Rudy!" chant that quickly goes stadium-wide. The offensive for the Fighting Irish ignores the coach's orders for a victory formation play and instead scores another touchdown. Finally, on the final kickoff, the coach lets Rudy play with the defensive team. He stays in for the final play of the game, sacks the opposing quarterback, and is carried off on the shoulders of his teammates.

All of this makes one wonder what Rudy could have done if he had been allowed more time on the field playing football. He overcame almost every obstacle a wanna-be football player could encounter, and yet, when given the chance, he achieved success. All it took was for him to get into the game.

In the same way, if you're gonna win, you gotta get in the game. Are you benching yourself because of health issues? Are you sitting there because you are too fat to get up and join the game of life? Is your idea of exercise lifting the weight of a fork full of food to your mouth? Face it: when it comes to your health, no one is making you sit on the bench but you. You can never win the fitness game just sitting there doing nothing. You can never achieve health and wholeness unless you fight inertia and get in the game.

Obesity, Health and Sexuality

The *Harvard Men's Health Watch*, the online bulletin of the Harvard Medical School, published a frightening article titled "Obesity: Unhealthy and Unmanly" in March 2011 that provides insight into why it is so critical for men to "get into the game." Shockingly, the study found that at present, *two-thirds* of all Americans need to lose weight. More frightening is the fact that obesity and lack of exercise kill about 1,000 Americans *every day*. According to the article, if present trends continue, obesity will soon overtake smoking as the leading preventable cause of death in the United States. You heard me right—preventable! Even though obesity affects both males and females, it affects men very differently and takes a particular toll on male hormones, sexuality and prostate health. If that isn't enough to scare you, obesity also increases the risks of a heart attack, stroke, hypertension, high cholesterol, diabetes, gallstones, cancer, osteoarthritis, obstructive sleep apnea, fatty liver and depression.

You probably already knew that obesity can cause the illnesses listed above, but let's talk about some of the lesser-known consequences.

- **Obesity and testosterone:** Obesity lowers testosterone levels. In a 2007 study of 1,667 men aged 40 and above, researchers found that each *one-point increase* in BMI was associated with a *two-percent decrease* in testosterone. Another study showed that a four-inch increase in waist size increased a man's odds of having a low testosterone level by 75 percent. Waist circumference was the strongest single predictor of developing symptoms of testosterone deficiency.

- **Erectile dysfunction and reproductive function:** Men with erectile dysfunction (ED) often blame low testosterone levels, but even when these levels are normal, men who are obese have an increased risk of ED. A Harvard study found that a man with a 42-inch waist is twice as likely to develop ED than a man with a 32-inch waist. In a Massachusetts study, researchers found that weight loss can improve these types of issues in overweight men with ED. In a study conducted by Italian scientists, researchers found that more than 30 percent of the 110 obese men who had followed a diet and exercise program in the study *corrected their ED without medication.* Those who lost the most weight enjoyed the greatest benefit. Other studies have linked obesity to low sperm counts and reduced sperm motility, which impair fertility in men.

- **Kidney stones:** Kidney stones are extremely painful, and they strike men twice as often as women. High BMIs and large waist circumference are both linked to an increased risk of kidney stones. According to a Harvard study, men who gain more than 35 pounds after age 21 are 39 percent more likely to develop stones than men who remain lean. Men of average height who weigh more than 220 pounds are 44 percent more likely to have stones than those who weigh less than 150 pounds. Studies from Europe and Asia show that the reason for this is because overweight people dump excess amounts of calcium and other chemicals into their urine, where the chemicals form stones.

- **Prostate cancer:** Obesity increases blood volume, which dilutes PSA (prostate-specific antigen) levels in the blood. This phenomenon makes it harder for doctors to use PSA measurements to detect prostate cancer in overweight guys. But that's not all. Obesity also has an adverse effect on the biology of prostate cancer. Research shows that extra body fat increases a man's risk of developing prostate cancer; in fact, an American Cancer Society study determined that being severely obese increases risk by *34 percent*. Obesity also increases the odds that prostate cancer will spread beyond the gland, and it also makes relapse after treatment more likely. Furthermore, obesity boosts a man's chance of developing urinary incontinence after a radical prostatectomy operation.[1]

Well, there you have it—an identification of some of the health crises men are facing today. These are just a few of the problems obesity causes, and many men aren't even aware of these problems—and don't even know they are at risk. But it doesn't have to be this way. You don't have to die an early death. You don't have to destroy your knees and your legs by packing too much weight. You don't have to deal with the illnesses and diseases mentioned above. There is hope. Remember, these things can be prevented. You can change your way of life to get better health and a better quality of life. You can have more energy. You can lose the excess weight. You can be around to see your kids and their kids grow up. In the rest of this book, I will tell you how.

Check Up

Big Belly = No Sex

There is significant evidence in the medical literature that obese and overweight men have poorer sexual function than their normal-weight counterparts. This is evidenced by the fact that obese men were 2½ times more likely to have erection problems than their non-obese counterparts. Although it is unknown whether this is caused by the weight itself or the associated medical problems (such as hypertension, high cholesterol, lower testosterone, diabetes, arterial disease or the medications necessary for these conditions), obesity is an important contributing factor to erectile dysfunction. Furthermore, a sedentary lifestyle, defined as spending three or more hours watching TV or being on the Internet all day, is also associated with erectile dysfunction.[2]

Are You Ready for Some Football?

For me, football was a way of life, and it was as natural for me as breathing. I began my college football career at Liberty University in 1976, where I was a starter all four years as an offensive tackle. I was responsible for blocking for the quarterback and running backs. Several small colleges and universities had recruited me, but I chose to attend the greatest university of all—Liberty University in Lynchburg, Virginia!

When I played for Liberty in the 1970s, the university was young but rapidly developing. At that time, it was moving up from the NCAA D-3 to the NCAA D-2 level. By my senior year in 1979, we were burying D-3 teams and dominating every D-2 team we played. We ended the year with a 9-1-1- record. That was the best winning percentage in Liberty University football history—a record that has stood for more than 34 years.

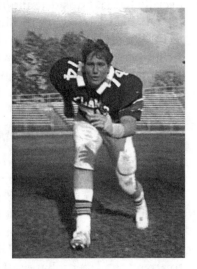

I was a specialty player at six-foot four-inches and a "blindside" left tackle. Not every lineman could do what I did. In passing situations, my job was critical in protecting our All-American quarterback, Glenn Inverso. (Glenn went on to play with the New York Jets.)

One of my teammates, Roy Jones, was a scruffy utility lineman who got the call when injuries occurred. During our senior year, he played center, guard, tackle and even tight end when we shifted to an unbalanced line. He pushed me, and I pushed him. I will always cherish one newspaper article I read about Jones and me and a huge six-foot, seven-inch, 365-pound defensive lineman we faced named Ernie White, who later on became a member of the Dallas Cowboys. The article, which I framed and today have hanging on my wall, always reminds me of how much I love the game of football and how much I enjoyed playing it with my teammates.

Two of my teammates themselves went on to play professional football, but I didn't even look in that direction. I knew God was calling me into full-time Christian ministry. My football scholarship was a means to an end. It provided a way for me to attend college, play the game I loved, and get equipped for the ministry I would one day have. It was a win, win, win!

At the end of my college football career, I was in the best shape of my life. I was exercising regularly, lifting weights and running. I really didn't have to watch what I ate, because whatever calories I took in I burned on the field or during practice. I felt great and looked great!

As I walked off the field that last game during my senior year, I vividly remember feeling exhausted. I was worn out . . . and burned out. I loved football, but I hated the practice and endless hours of physical training and exercise. The sport had been a focal part of my life for years, and I was tired of it. I had begun playing in a youth football league at the age of eight, and I had played every year until I graduated from Liberty. That's a lot of running, weight lifting and wind sprints—the kind of exercise I especially hated. I dreaded and hated practice, and I really didn't like running. I was sick of coaches yelling at me. I was ready to move from the field to the stands, where I could watch the game I loved so much.

It wasn't that I stopped loving the game. In fact, I'm a huge fan of the Washington Redskins. I was just ready to move on to another chapter in my life and do something different. I thought, *Thank God this is over!*

New Wife, New Life!

I met my wife, Debbie, toward the end of my freshman year of college. We dated all through college and were married on December 15, 1979. Unfortunately, like most men, after I was married I felt as if I no longer had to worry about impressing anyone with the way I looked. After all, I had a beautiful wife, so I could check that one off the list.

I graduated from Liberty University in the spring of 1980 and went on to attend the Liberty Baptist Theological Seminary. I graduated with my Master's Degree in counseling in the spring of 1982. During this time, Debbie and I were settling into our new life together. We were excited about the future and about starting a new chapter of our lives.

We left Lynchburg, Virginia, and headed to northern Virginia in the summer of 1982. I had the degrees, I had the girl, and I now had a new goal: to start a brand-new church plant right outside Washington, DC. I knew this was a risky move, as the statistics at the time stated that only 1 out of 10 new churches would survive any length of time.

The good news is that we beat the odds! After a lot of hard work and determination, my ministry grew. Over a period of 30 years, we were able to grow a successful ministry in this difficult area. The bad news is that I grew right along with the ministry. While everything seemed to be going great in my life, with my beautiful wife and then the addition of three awesome kids, there was one huge issue with which I had never dealt. Even though I had hung up my jersey, pads and cleats and said goodbye to playing football, I was still eating like a football player. This time, however, I didn't have a coach yelling and screaming at me to get my butt down the field and run sprints. I no longer had to impress anyone, and I didn't have to keep physically fit to stay on the team. So, as you can imagine, I began to grow and grow and grow, until I reached my heaviest weight of 340 pounds. My six-pack soon became a keg!

Keeping a Deadly Promise

So, how could a football player go from being in the best shape of his life to becoming obese? I blame it all on one deadly promise I made to myself the day I walked off the field after that last game at Liberty. You see, I didn't just say, "Thank God this is over." Instead, I made a promise to myself that I would *never* exercise or run again! Nobody was going to tell me to sprint, lift weights or do blocking drills. There were a lot of promises I regretfully broke over the years, but this was one promise that I kept—and I kept it wholeheartedly! I didn't exercise, and I kept eating whatever and whenever I wanted. I became a glutton! I ended up in a place I never expected to be—in the wrong end zone—and weighing almost one-fifth of a ton.

The truth was that I was a hypocrite. I had no problem standing in the pulpit preaching to my congregation on every sin known to man while I trashed my body with food and diligently avoided exercise. I had no problem telling them that they needed to lay any idols or gods in their life at the feet of Jesus and serve and glorify Him with their whole being while I lived a double life and served my own god. My belly was my god, and the food I put into it was my idol. I reflected Paul's words in Philippians 3:19: "Whose end is destruction, whose god is their belly, and whose glory is in their shame—who set their mind earthly things." I even remember hearing a respected and well-known pastor talking about health and thinking to myself, *Why is this guy wasting his time talking about that? We have more important things to deal with.*

I was living for myself and the lusts of my flesh. At 340 pounds, I was battling diabetes, high blood pressure and high cholesterol. You would think all that would be enough of a wake-up call, but I wanted an easy quick-fix solution to these serious problems I had created. I would walk into my doctor's office and say things like, "I'm busy . . . you're busy . . . so let's make this quick. Just write me a prescription, and we'll both be on our way." I was looking for a pill or a potion that would make it all go away. I wanted something easy that required little to no work on my part.

If I Don't Get Up, I'm Gonna Die!

I had no one to blame for my health situation but myself. I was reaping what I had sown all those years since I had played my last football game. My wakeup call came when I finally realized that I was killing myself slowly with a knife and a fork and an ice cream spoon. The thought of heading to an early grave was terrifying. My health had deteriorated to the point that this was a possibility. I knew that if I didn't do something, I was going to die. What would happen to my wife, my children, and my ministry? I was so sick and tired of being sick and tired, and the thought of having to take prescription after prescription for the rest of my life was no longer acceptable.

This was not the way I had imagined my life would be on that day I walked off the football field with such hope for the future. I had been so young, healthy and full of dreams. I had been ready to take risks, live dangerously, have fun doing it and prove that I could make it in a difficult area of ministry when all the statistics were against me. For me, failure was not an option. I dreamed of whom I would be—the type of impact I would have on my kids, my grandchildren, my community, my ministry. But in the physical condition I was in, I now doubted whether I would even meet my grandchildren and have the opportunity to invest in them.

I was taking risks all right—risks with my health; risks that displeased my Creator; risks that could kill me. What type of impact would I leave behind if I dropped dead of a heart attack because I was too fat? That was not how I wanted to leave this life. It was not how I wanted to be remembered. I had to do something, and I wasn't sure what that something was. I just knew I had to change. I had become a "la-Z-y bum" sitting in the La-Z-Boy. I had to say to myself, *Get off the couch, you lazy bum!*

Can you relate to my story? Have health issues benched you and forced you to watch life pass by instead of enjoying being healthy and productive? In the following pages, I am going to walk you through how I went from the couch to getting back in the game and to winning again. You will also hear from men just like you who took action and were successful in making positive changes in the area of their health.

Life is far too short and precious, and you are way too valuable and important to be just sitting around. Don't choose death . . . choose life! You are on God's team, and He created you to honor and glorify Him with your life and your body. Know that you can do all things through Christ who strengthens you (see Philippians 4:13). Keep reading, and see just how much of a miracle you really are.

Keith Brown
Gets Back in the Game

LOST 45 POUNDS

Before	After
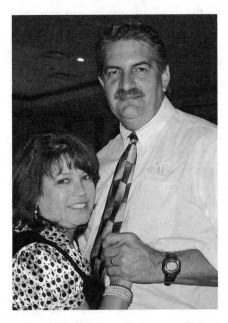	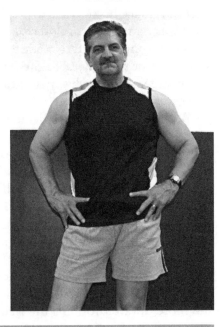

Over the years, I made many attempts at transformation. I'd say, "Okay, I'll start on Monday." Monday would come, and then Tuesday, and then by Wednesday so many obstacles had come up that I would push doing any transforming off until the next week. Talk about denial. As I looked into the mirror each morning, I saw myself as a younger, healthier and more fit man than the reflection actually portrayed.

I used to think that positive change begins in the mind, but I have come to realize that it starts in the heart. For me, this was the hardest part of change—moving the decision from my head to my heart. I had been an athlete in my younger days and was always in shape, so admitting I needed help was somewhat humbling. It was a blow to my ego. Understand that my idea of being "in shape" back then was being able to play sports, not get injured, and still be able to brag about eating anything I wanted without having to worry about getting fat. *That's not something I'll ever have to worry about,* I told myself. Talk about having to eat crow.

As the years rolled on, my metabolism slowed to a crawl, but my appetite maintained its momentum. It was not until I found a roll of film in the "junk drawer" and had it developed that I realized how much I had let myself go and how bad I looked. Among the pictures was a photo of my dad and me taken just before he had his third open-heart surgery, this time to replace his aorta. Although he did fine during the surgery, his heart was damaged from previous heart attacks and bad eating. It was just not strong enough to restart and keep pumping on its own, and he went on to be with the Lord the same day as the surgery. I knew I had to take charge of my situation and take care of myself to be better able to take care of my family.

Because I am a large individual, at first the weight I was putting on was not noticeable on the outside, but it was taking its toll on the inside. My family has a history of heart problems, high cholesterol, diabetes and high blood pressure, and it hit me all at once that I was doing just what I needed to do in order to find myself up to my neck in some of these same problem areas. I didn't like it. I had gone from being active to a way-too-busy-to-exercise person, and the weight had begun to show. I found myself at the bottom of the fitness abyss at 294 pounds, 25.6 percent body fat, with a cholesterol level at 194.

My energy had gone down, and my physical limitations were beginning to take hold and control my activities. I found myself looking more and more toward dropping my recliner into "third gear" and waiting for "tired" to take over. I would watch some of the activities around the neighborhood—pick-up basketball, men's softball, tennis—and though my heart was still playing, my body could not. I was in the stands due to my health and weight. It hurt.

I have participated in many challenges since then and have had success in most of them. My accomplishments allowed me to appear on the Montel Williams show as a fitness challenge winner. I appeared in a Bowflex infomercial that ran nationally for about a year. I won a trip to Jamaica as a result of a fitness challenge, and I was able to participate in the Olympic Torch Relay for the 2002 Winter Olympics in Salt Lake City, Utah.

In spite of all the successes, I still had a feeling of emptiness. I had questions. *Why am I doing this? I know it is a "lifestyle" change, and I have made that change, so now what?* I found the answer in the book *Bod4God: Four Keys to Weight Loss* by Pastor Steve Reynolds.[3] I realized that not only could I live a healthy lifestyle, but also what I do, how I did it and with whom I shared the program could be a prevalent motivating factor for my own health. I could use the book and the Losing to Live weight loss competition program to share, teach and guide others toward a positive change.

A healthy life is inspiring. It has given me a new drive and, more importantly, a means to navigate troubled waters and "right my ship" before it capsizes. *Bod4God* has shown me how to have physical change while integrating biblical concepts and heart change. I have stayed in pretty good shape for a number of years now. My current weight is 249, my body fat is at 14 percent, and my cholesterol level is at 128. Not bad for a 55 year old guy.

But even better than what I have done is what God has done through Pastor Steve Reynolds. Since finding the book and meeting Pastor Reynolds, the Cathedral of Praise Church has sponsored two different Losing to Live weight loss competitions here in Charleston, South Carolina. We started with 210 people in the first program, and by following the guidelines from *Bod4God*, our group lost 1,765 pounds. Our second program began with 119 people, and we collectively lost 1,245 pounds.

We love *Bod4God* and the Losing to Live program, and we thank God and Pastor Steve for inspiring us to accomplish our goals.

Man Up

Eat Up: Watch Your Portion Size

This week, it's time to seriously start thinking about portion control and how much you are eating. Your stomach is approximately the size of your fist, so why are you eating the size of your head? Start by being intentional when putting food on your plate, and make it a point to limit your portions. Remember to put your fork down between each bite, chew thoroughly, and take a few deep breaths before you put more food in your mouth. Remember that it takes 20 minutes for your brain to register that you are full, so take your time and savor every bite.*

Pump Up: Walk the Walk

Man Up! It's time to take action, and it's time to get moving. Exercise is movement—the more you move, the more you lose. So this week, think of little ways to intentionally move your body. Your feet were made for walking, so start by walking two to three times this week (10 to 15 minutes per outing). You can even take your phone calls as you do so to pass the time. As you walk, make sure to monitor your breathing—if you are breathing too hard to talk, you are walking too fast. Keep a log of the days you walked and the actual time you did the exercise. If this gets too easy, do a light jog/brisk walk, or increase the minutes. Do this every week from here on out and, as you progress, add an additional day or increase the minutes.**

---

* My thanks to Nancy Parlette, MS, for her contribution to the Man Up: Eat Up sections included in this book. You can learn more about her and her book *The Busy Mom's Ten Minute Guide to a Healthy, Happy Family* at www.nancyparlette.com.

** My thanks to Cedric Bryant, Certified Health and Fitness Professional NASM, IFA, CPT, for his contribution to the Man Up: Pump Up sections included in this book. Note: be sure to consult your physician before starting any exercise program.

Reflection and Discussion Questions

1. What are some of the common excuses guys make about their sedentary lifestyle?

   _____

   _____

   _____

   _____

2. What has been keeping you on the couch and out of the game of living a healthy and productive life?

   _____

   _____

   _____

   _____

3. Now that you have read this chapter, you know the statistics about what happens to overweight and under-exercised men. How do you think your health has been impacted by your current lifestyle?

   _____

   _____

   _____

   _____

4. In this chapter, the author talks about a deadly promise that he regretted making to himself to stop exercising. What choices have you made that have negatively affected your health?

   _____

   _____

   _____

   _____

   _____

5. Can you relate to Paul's words Philippians 3:19? In what ways has your belly become your god?

_____

_____

_____

_____

6. Philippians 4:13 says you can do all things through Christ. In what ways do you need Christ to strengthen you as you begin to get off the couch and get in the game?

_____

_____

_____

_____

MY PERSONAL GAME PLAN FOR

GETTING IN SHAPE

*Beloved, I pray that you may prosper in all things
and be in health, just as your soul prospers.*

3 JOHN 2

This book is about **ACTION** and about **DOING**! In the spaces below, record what actions you are going to take to improve your health this week.

Aware—I will do the following to show I am aware of my current physical condition and that my body matters to God:

_____

_____

_____

_____

_____

Commit—I will do the following to commit to living a disciplined life and to winning over temptation:

_____

_____

_____

_____

_____

Transform—This is how I will transform the way I think and live:

_____

_____

_____

_____

_____

Incorporate—I will incorporate these healthy eating habits and exercise into my daily life:

_____

_____

_____

_____

_____

Organize—This is how I will organize a team of people to help me win:

_____

_____

_____

_____

_____

Navigate—This is my action plan for healthy living and navigating my way to leaving a lasting legacy:

_____

_____

_____

_____

_____

Chapter 2

Your Body Matters to God

Do you not know that your body is the temple of the Holy Spirit who is in you, whom you have from God, and you are not your own?
1 CORINTHIANS 6:19

"Gentlemen, this is a football." These were the first words the players of the Green Bay Packers heard from Vince Lombardi, their legendary coach, on the first day of practice. Think about it: These men had probably played football for many years. They wouldn't have made it to the pros if they didn't understand the game and how it was played. They certainly knew what a football was. So why would Coach Lombardi start with these five simple words? Why would he then show them the layout of the field and explain the rules of the game and the roles and responsibilities of the players? The reason is because he wanted to bring them back to the *basics*. He wanted them to be aware of what they were doing and why they were doing it.

In the previous chapter, I told you my story. Now I want to bring you back to the basics and make you aware of what the Bible says about your body. So I say to you, "Gentlemen, this is your body."

Don't Get Sad, Get Mad!

Right now, when you look in the mirror and see what you have become, you probably feel pretty discouraged. You probably feel paralyzed by your current physical condition and unable to see how you could ever change. What you need to remember is that you are miraculous, custom-made and lovingly crafted by God. There is more to you than what you see on the outside. So instead of getting sad, it is time to get mad—mad enough to resolve to begin making changes right now.

A football player who carries the ball toward his goal line while looking back over his shoulder is likely to get knocked down. In the same way, you can't make any serious progress toward your goal while focusing on past mistakes. It's time to put your eye on the end result and focus all your energy on moving forward. While it is all right to learn about the negative and destructive things you have done to your body, it is not all right to allow those things to prevent you from moving forward. You must dump the negative, start thinking about the positive, and develop a plan that will take you where you want to go in the future.

One of the first things I did when I stepped onto the field of living a healthy life was to examine how I was living. *I quickly realized that my decisions had not only negatively impacted me but had also negatively impacted my entire family.* Because I did most of the cooking and grocery shopping at our house, I controlled the kinds of food my family ate. My choices with regard to food and health had trickled down to the people whom I loved the most. This hit me hard. I had dedicated a lot of time and attention to making sure they were spiritually healthy, but I had completely failed in making sure they were physically healthy. I deeply regretted the fact that I had not been a good example to my family in this area. I felt as if I were a lousy husband and father.

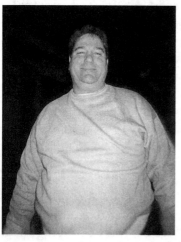

However, instead of allowing these feelings to paralyze me and keep me from moving toward a goal of healthy living, I decided to take action. Sure, I had made some poor choices, and those choices had consequences. But I could start making better choices immediately, and those good choices would produce good consequences for me and my loved ones.

In many ways, I had become a "temple trasher." In John 2:12-16, we read the story of how one day Jesus went to the Temple to worship and there found moneychangers and merchants selling their goods and wares inside the Temple area. These men had trashed God's holy place and turned it into a den of thieves, just as I was trashing my body. Like Jesus, I had to get angry and start turning over the tables in my life where I was buying into the lies Satan was telling me—lies that I didn't have to eat

42

right, didn't have to exercise, and didn't have to take care of my body. I had said for years that I wanted to be like Jesus, and now it was time to start living what I claimed.

I had lost sight of the fact that in 1 Corinthians 6:19, Paul says, "Do you not know that your body is the temple of the Holy Spirit, who is in you, whom you received from God?" My body was the Temple of God—the place where the Holy Spirit resides. How dare I trash His temple? I love how Coach Joe Gibbs, former coach of my favorite team, the Washington Redskins, puts it:

> Me? A temple? Yep. As a believer in Jesus Christ, your heart is a place of residence for the Spirit of God. Your body is a sanctuary, a special piece of construction designed to be treated with the same kind of care and decorum you exercise when you're at church. So for the same reason you don't scarf down nachos during worship service or wear your lawn-mowing clothes to Sunday school, you should treat your physical body with respect, honor and a real sense of worth.[1]

Have you ever thought about the fact that the Holy Spirit sits down with you at every meal? He is there every time you put food in your mouth. This fact certainly got my attention. I needed to take care of my body—this miracle of life that God created. I needed to have a new appreciation for the gift it truly is. I needed to realize that I was trashing the temple of God and do something about it.

Skinny Fat Guys

Maybe you are one of those guys who aren't obese or terribly overweight, and you don't feel that you are trashing God's temple. You are what I call one of those "skinny fat" people. Even though you aren't significantly overweight, you lead a sedentary, unhealthy lifestyle of doing what you want and eating what you want. If this fits you, know that this book is for you just as much as it is for the guy sitting there with 100 pounds or more to lose. While you could weigh the appropriate amount for your height, you could still be a walking time bomb just waiting to go off. You could still be trashing your temple with the unhealthy food that you are consuming and your refusal to get active and exercise. You still have a responsibility to God to treat His temple with honor, and you still need to get healthy! But don't take it from me. Listen to my friend Glenn Schlarman and consider whether you are "skinny fat" like he was.

I've always been competitive by nature. When I entered the Losing to Live weight loss competition, I lost 17 pounds—but it wasn't about weight, it was about health. When I was employed, I used to eat only one meal a day. When I retired, I began to eat three meals a day rather than one, and my only exercise was yard work, which I did only seasonally. I suffered with acid reflux and was taking medicine for that condition.

When the Losing to Live competition came, my wife wanted to participate. At that time there was a doctor attending my church who checked everyone's blood, and my triglycerides were so high that he couldn't get a cholesterol reading. I have a family history of heart attacks, stroke and high everything, so this got my attention. Although I didn't do anything drastic, I began paying attention to living healthier.

My clothes still fit, so I didn't worry. But when I heard Pastor Steve say that our stomach was the size of our fist, I realized that I was eating meals the size of Mohammed Ali's fist inside a boxing glove. I used to lie down after a meal, so I stopped doing that. I stopped eating late into the evening, cut down my portion sizes, changed snacks (an apple instead of chips), and drank more water. I started walking a couple of miles a day. I became healthier and got rid of the purple pill I was taking.

Men are supposed to be leaders: at home, at work, and in society. Every excuse they use about overeating or not exercising is evidence that they are not leading but following someone or something else. If we men were to assume the responsibility we find in Scripture for how we should live our lives, we probably wouldn't have as many health problems—at least not self-induced health problems.

Check Up

Big Belly = Death Risk

According to the National Institute of Health, obesity and overweight are the second leading cause of preventable death in the United States, after tobacco use. Three hundred thousand deaths per year are caused by the obesity epidemic,[2] and obesity is associated with a higher chance of dying from heart disease or cancer.[3] In other words, if you have heart disease or cancer and you are overweight, you have a higher chance of dying from these diseases. In men, a BMI greater than 26.5 was most strongly associated with cardiovascular mortality. (To figure your BMI, refer to appendix B.)

There will be people in your office who will encourage you to make unhealthy choices. While friends and colleagues would never encourage an alcoholic to drink, they will pester you to join the party and eat the unhealthy food they have brought into the workplace. If you have friends and colleagues who are not fully supportive of your goals for a healthier lifestyle, speak with them about it. If that doesn't work, it's time to reexamine your friendships. As Dave Ramsey says, "If you can't change your friends, change your friends." This doesn't mean that you should shift the blame to them—shifting blame at best is unbecoming, and at worst cowardly and unbiblical. Take responsibility for your own actions, deal with them, and surround yourself with people who support your decision.

When I started changing my lifestyle, I felt pressure from others. I felt they were watching and waiting for me to fail. But I couldn't allow that to stop me from pressing on. I understood that healthy living is a long process, and I knew I had to pace myself. So let me encourage you. When you begin leading a healthier lifestyle, take it incrementally so you can sustain your changes. Remember that you're hitting singles, not home runs. In the beginning you might have trouble, but if you keep going, it will work.

Remember Ted Williams? He was the last baseball player to hit over .400 in a single season. That was more than 70 years ago. His career average was a whopping .344. Think about it: in his best year, he failed 60 percent of the time; and for his career, he failed almost 70 percent of the time. But did he quit, make excuses or blame others? Nope, he kept on going and today, of course, he is in the Baseball Hall of Fame.

You can be a Hall of Famer too—a Hall of Famer in gaining a new lifestyle of healthy living.

The Bible, the Best Health Book!

For years I preached that the Bible had all the answers for life—all the information one could need to be successful—but I really didn't know what the Bible had to say about our bodies and our health. I knew that Paul said in 1 Corinthians 6:19 that our bodies were the temple of the Holy Spirit, and I knew that God had created us, but I had never taken the time to learn how I should care for His creation. So I started studying and found that the word "body" is mentioned 179 times in the *King James Version*. That surprised me. Then I remembered Paul's words in Colossians 1:16: "All things were created through him and for him." Wow! I mattered to God!

I think we already know this in the back of our minds, but do we really believe it? Do we live as if we matter to God? Furthermore, because we matter to God, He has given us the best health book we could ever have—the Bible! But have we taken the time to read it? We have been given all the instructions we need to care for this miracle body, but we will never learn what we need to know unless we open it.

Now, I know you probably hate the word "instructions." Perhaps you have been forced to put together one of those bikes or dollhouses on Christmas Eve so they would be ready for the big surprise on Christmas Day. Maybe you spent hours and hours trying to figure out how all the pieces fit together, and when you were finished you had extra parts that didn't seem to fit anywhere. Of course, you never looked at the instructions. Why would you need them? After all, you are a man! It's likely you stayed up all night doing what might have taken you half the time if you had followed the instructions and made slow progress toward your goal.

It is only by reading God's Word that we can discover His instruction—His plan—for our lives. The world's idea of how to get healthy has a lot to do with quick fixes, pills and potions. These are not God's ways of getting healthy. The world wants us to believe that instead of being God's creation, we evolved; and that instead of honoring God with our bodies, we can do whatever we want with them. On the playing field of life, the interference we have to run is that God's truths are contrary to everything the world wants us to believe. God's ideas are different, and they are much better than what the world has to offer to us.

When I took the time to carefully study what the Bible has to say about our bodies, I found two things that really hit home with me: (1) We were made *by* God, and (2) we were made *for* God. Let that sink in for a minute: God really cares about us, and He wants us to live a healthy and abundant life. Let's take a closer look at each of these principles.

1. We Were Made by God

God doesn't create junk. The human body is marvelous and miraculous, and God gave us everything we need to sustain life. The following is an impressive list of human body facts that show the wisdom and care of our Creator:

- A special region in the middle of the brain, called the periaqueductal gray, releases endorphins—natural pain-killers that are more powerful than morphine. Endorphins keep the body from going into shock.[4]

- Heat from the movement of our rapidly beating heart would kill us if it were not designed with a special lubricated bag, called the pericardial sac, which reduces friction.[5]

- Unlike the wires in a hardwired computer, our brain cells are constantly making new connections. The connections that are repeatedly used become stronger, while those that are unused can be lost in a process called pruning.[6]

- Amazingly, we are born with all the hair follicles we will ever have, and these follicles normally continue to produce hairs throughout our lives. As a person ages, some follicles that produce terminal hairs begin to replace them with almost invisible vellus hairs. So, we actually don't lose hairs as we get older—our hair just gets smaller.[7]

- Our lungs are so efficient that studies have shown that most people must lose nearly three-fourths of their lung tissue before serious respiratory difficulty develops. Our lungs have about 800 million alveolar air sacs.[8]

- The weight of the total blood circulated through our lungs each day is around eight tons.[9]

- The three small bones in the middle ear are known collectively as ossicles. They are the three smallest bones in the body (the smallest bone weighs .0001 ounces.) They are the only bones that never grow larger from the time of birth to old age.[10]

Wow! There is a Creator, and He took great care when creating us. As David writes in Psalm 139:13-17:

For You formed my inward parts;
    You covered me in my mother's womb.
I will praise You, for I am fearfully and wonderfully made;
    Marvelous are Your works,
    And that my soul knows very well.
My frame was not hidden from You,
    When I was made in secret,

And skillfully wrought in the lowest parts of the earth.
Your eyes saw my substance, being yet unformed.
 And in Your book they all were written,
 The days fashioned for me,
 when as yet there were none of them.
How precious also are Your thoughts to me, O God!
 How great is the sum of them!

You can't tell me that the amazing creation we are just happened by chance any more than you could tell me a football stadium just happened by chance (or that it evolved from a soccer field). Someone planned and created that stadium, and Someone planned and created the miracle that is us. And not only did God create us, but we are precious to Him. He loves us and cares about us. Perhaps right now because of the way you look you feel a sense of uselessness or unworthiness, but remember that the creation is always precious to the Creator.

2. We Were Made *for* God

As Christians, we understand that God is our creator, but we struggle with the fact that He needs to be in control of our bodies. In 1 Corinthians 6:19-20, after Paul tells us that our bodies are the temple of the Holy Spirit, he adds, "Do you not know that . . . you are not your own? For you were bought at a price. Therefore, glorify God in your body and in your spirit which are God's."

When we accepted Christ as our Savior and Lord, God moved in, and our bodies became His temple. We joined His franchise. He owns us. He paid the price to have us on His team, and He paid it in full when His Son, Jesus, left heaven, came to earth, lived a perfect and sinless life, suffered for our sin, was nailed to a cross and died.

Thankfully, that's not the end of the story. He was buried, and on the third day He rose from the grave to give us eternal life. In the same way that a football player cannot indulge in unhealthy food and fail to show up for training, we cannot eat what is unhealthy just because it tastes good or makes us feel better. We are part of God's team, and we must live like players on the greatest eternal team of all.

I Found the Secret

Let me give you the secret to weight loss that I found in the Bible. It's way simpler than the weight-loss pills advertised in men's health magazines, or the latest diet fad, or the surgery to reduce the size of your stomach. It's this: eat less and exercise more! It's just that easy.

Eat Less

Gluttony—the over-indulgence in anything to the point of waste—is a deadly sin. The secret of avoiding the sin of gluttony is to learn how to control your portions. Make a fist. That represents about the size of your stomach, and it's not going to take a lot to fill it. Now look at your head in a mirror. Many people eat a pile of food the size of their head. Sorry, pal, but that's just too much for that fist-sized stomach. You have to eat less, and you have to eat healthier.

Let me ask you a question: Are you eating for your health or for your happiness? This is an important question, because people view food and their food choices by what makes them happy. I know this is true because it's what I did—and it resulted in my weighing 340 pounds and having to deal with high blood pressure, high cholesterol and diabetes. Men, we have got to get it through our skulls that eating isn't about whether or not it makes us happy but about whether it makes us healthy.

The good news is that if you keep eating what makes you healthy, before long it will also make you happy. Here's how it works. At first, the change will feel like a huge sacrifice. But before long you will say, "This isn't bad." Later, you will say, "I love this!" Before you know it, thinking about the stuff you used to eat will make you feel sick. Your body will reject it.

In Deuteronomy 8:7, I love the way God tells the Israelites that He is bringing them "into a good land." This is how He describes a good land: "A land of brooks of water, of fountains and springs, that flow out of valleys and hills; a land of wheat and barley, of vines and fig trees and pomegranates, a land of olive oil and honey" (verses 7-8). It's not Superbowl food—potato chips, barbequed wings, ice cream, cookies and gallons of soda. The food God describes is living food, and He calls it good. While you might not think that what the Bible describes is very manly, just how manly is it to suffer from diseases and weight-related physical conditions?

When I weighed 340 pounds, Proverbs 23:2 always bothered me: "Put a knife to your throat if you are a man given to appetite." I would quickly skip over the verse and try to ignore it. The fact was that I didn't understand what it meant. Sure, I knew I was a man given to appetite, and I knew I didn't like knives (particularly around my throat), but I didn't understand that it was speaking about gluttony. It is serious business when you have a gluttony problem, and it calls for action. In other words, the writer of this proverb is telling the glutton, "Change your life!"

Exercise More

The other half of the secret I uncovered is that God designed us to be physically active. Genesis 2:15 says, "The Lord God took the man and put him in the Garden of Eden." To do what? Sit around and eat? No, to work. To tend the Garden and keep it.

Do you know anything about yard work and keeping a garden? It's work! God said to Adam, "Buddy, you are going to work here. You are going to move. You are going to exercise. You are going to tend and keep this garden." After mankind's fall into sin, the work became even harder. Adam had to till the ground and hoe out the thistles, briars and weeds. From the very beginning, God expected us to be physically active.

Exercise means movement. It means getting your body in gear, letting out the clutch, and moving forward. It may mean going to a gym. It may mean taking the steps rather than the elevator. It may mean parking your car as far away as possible from your destination so you can walk to it. It means getting up off the couch—or out of the La-Z-Boy—and moving. We will be unpacking these two secrets in more depth throughout the book.

Do You Want to Be Successful?

"Success" is a word that gets most men's attention, but it is one not mentioned often the Bible. One place we find this word is in Joshua 1:8, which states, "This Book of the Law shall not depart from your mouth, but you shall meditate in it day and night, that you may observe to do according to all that is written in it. For then you will make your way prosperous, and then you will have good success" (Joshua 1:8). This is God's formula for success: meditating on the Book of the Law (the Bible) both day and night.

If you are going to succeed at anything in life—especially when it comes to your health and losing weight—you must start reading the Bible. It is from the Bible that you gain knowledge, inspiration and support. It was in the pages of the Bible that I found the formula for a better body and a healthy lifestyle. Here is what the Bible taught me:

1. I had to adopt a new lifestyle, not a weight-loss plan.
2. I had to honor God with my whole being—God wanted to use me and could only do that by using my hands, feet, mind and body.

3. I had to become motivated to live a healthier life by incorporating new healthy habits that would bring about change.
4. I had to stop choosing foods that were killing me.
5. I had to get off the couch and become physically active.
6. I had to have God's help and the help of other strugglers on the same path of life.
7. I had to begin taking "Small Steps to Life."

Once I implemented these changes, I lost more than 120 pounds. I stopped taking all medications. I no longer had diabetes, high cholesterol or high blood pressure.

Something is wrong with our society's complicated plans for weight loss. If those plans worked, we wouldn't need to have thousands of books, diet products, TV shows and magazines telling us over and over how to lose weight. So instead of turning to those plans, why not try God's plan found in His health book—the Bible? What do you have to lose at this point? Nothing!

I'm convinced that you will find His way is the best way—the way that will lead not only to lasting results in the areas of health and wellness but also to a deeper and more lasting relationship with God. So let me urge you to do as I've done and turn God's health book into your playbook and commit to change your lifestyle from unhealthy to healthy. Read on, and I'll show you how.

Jeff Townsend's
Narrow Escape

LOST 261 POUNDS

Before	After
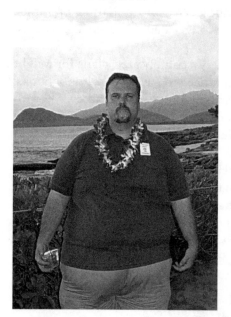	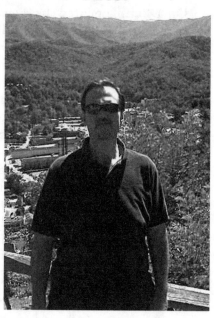

From my childhood, I always struggled with my weight. I developed unhealthy behavior patterns early in life, and I grew up being told "finish your plate." Well, I managed to finish my plate—and then some. By the time I was a sophomore in high school, I weighed more than 300 pounds. I did not know how to lose weight the right way, so when I was a junior in high school, I went on a "no eating" diet. I ate nothing but tuna, coffee and weight-loss supplements. By the end of my senior year in high school I weighed 165 pounds. Physically, I looked good; however, emotionally, I was a wreck. I became a border-line bulimic. I didn't understand the importance of caring for my body.

After high school, I enlisted in the US Navy and was stationed on the USS Nimitz. I worked in a fire suit on the flight deck in extreme heat for

16 hours a day. Keeping the weight off was not a problem, and I weighed 165 pounds throughout my military career. Still, I never learned the proper way to maintain my weight. Not eating seemed to be the best way to keep the weight off.

After leaving the military, I slowly started putting the weight back on. By 1992, I was back up to 240 pounds. I discovered I had diverticulitis, and doctors had to remove 70 percent of my colon. They had no explanation as to why I had this disease, as it usually occurs in elderly people, and I did not discover the cause for years. Eventually, I discovered is that people who are bulimic or anorexic—as I was—can do severe damage to their colons. I had to wear a colostomy bag for two years, and I had six operations before the surgeon could connect my colon again. During this two-year period, I went through bouts of severe depression and gained another 60 pounds. In a 10-year time span, I managed to put back on all of the weight of my high school years.

During 1994–2008, I went on a dozen different diets to lose weight. I would lose 50 pounds and then gain back 70. Eventually, in 2008 when my weight peaked at 461 pounds, both my wife and I decided to have gastric bypass surgery. We had heard nothing but positive things about the surgery, and we thought it was the most effective way to lose weight. Have you ever said, "If I knew then what I know now"?

I went in for surgery on November 3, 2008. My surgery lasted nine hours, and at first it appeared to be a success. But then, on day two of my recovery, my temperature spiked, and tests revealed that I had a leak. I became septic and underwent 17 surgeries during the next 43 days. I was placed in the intensive care unit and put into a medically induced coma. It was a day-to-day process to see if I was going to make it. Ultimately, I was in the hospital 91 days and in rehab for six months. You don't know what you have until it is gone. I had to learn to walk all over again.

Since my initial bypass surgery in November 2008, I have had a total of 19 surgeries. The last surgery took place this past January when doctors discovered I had a hole in my small intestine caused by a suture that had punctured it. It happened when I got out of my car—my stomach ruptured, and food and liquid leaked into a pocket under my skin above the abdomen. Even today, I do not have an abdominal wall; and therefore I am limited in how I can exercise.

A friend one day told me about Pastor Steve and his success with *Bod4God* and the Losing to Live weight loss competition. I had known Steve years back when he baptized my wife, and he had performed the marriage ceremony for one of my dearest friends more than 20 years ago. Only

God knew that we would be brought together through the one common thing we both struggled with our entire life—food!

I know without a shadow of a doubt that I am here today because of our Lord and Savior. He saved me. I am also here to serve as living proof that you cannot lose weight or maintain your weight loss without prayer and a support system. While gastric bypass surgery might cause you to lose weight, it will not change your mindset or help you exercise. In my case, it almost killed me. People who are considering this operation should understand all of the risks and the post-surgery effect it will have on their lives.

The Lord has convicted my heart to live the rest of my life serving Him and glorifying His name through helping others. I am blessed to be able to share my story with people who are struggling and help them as they work to lead a healthier life.

Man Up

Eat Up: Start with Water

Wake up with water. Drink an 8-ounce glass when you get up, and work up to half your body weight in ounces each day. In other words, if you weigh 200 pounds, drink 100 ounces of water each day. Every metabolic action in your body requires water, and drinking water will flush out the toxins that your body stores in fat. Drink 12 ounces of water whenever you think you are hungry and before meals. Most of the time, you will actually just be thirsty, so refreshing with water will help curb your food cravings.

Pump Up: Step It Up

Using your surroundings to get in a workout is a great way to minimize excuses for not being able to exercise. Find a set of stairs, and walk up and down them. Do this three times in five-minute increments with a 90-second rest between rounds. If this gets too easy, carry weights or grab a backpack and place some books in it to add resistance, or increase your tempo and speed.

Reflection and Discussion Questions

1. Where are you in your weight-loss journey? Are you discouraged? Frustrated? Sad? Angry? What changes do you plan to make?

   _____

   _____

   _____

   _____

   _____

2. Have you ever viewed the Bible as a health book? If so, what are some passages that come to mind when you think of it that way?

   _____

   _____

   _____

   _____

3. What is your take on the idea that you are made by God and for God?

   _____

   _____

   _____

   _____

   _____

   _____

4. If God made you and you are His prized creation, what do you think you can expect from Him in terms of help in your weight-loss battle?

   _____

   _____

   _____

   _____

5. Are you eating to make yourself healthy or happy? Why?

_____

_____

_____

_____

_____

6. In 1 Corinthians 6:19, Paul says that your body is the temple of the Holy Spirit. In what ways have you been a "temple trasher," and what will you do about it?

_____

_____

_____

_____

_____

MY PERSONAL GAME PLAN FOR

GETTING IN SHAPE

*Beloved, I pray that you may prosper in all things
and be in health, just as your soul prospers.*

3 JOHN 2

This book is about **ACTION** and about **DOING**! In the spaces below, record what actions you are going to take to improve your health this week.

Aware—I will do the following to show I am aware of my current physical condition and that my body matters to God:

_____
_____
_____
_____
_____

Commit—I will do the following to commit to living a disciplined life and to winning over temptation:

_____
_____
_____
_____
_____
_____

Transform—This is how I will transform the way I think and live:

_____
_____
_____
_____
_____

Incorporate—I will incorporate these healthy eating habits and exercise into my daily life:

_____

_____

_____

_____

_____

Organize—This is how I will organize a team of people to help me win:

_____

_____

_____

_____

_____

Navigate—This is my action plan for healthy living and navigating my way to leaving a lasting legacy:

_____

_____

_____

_____

_____

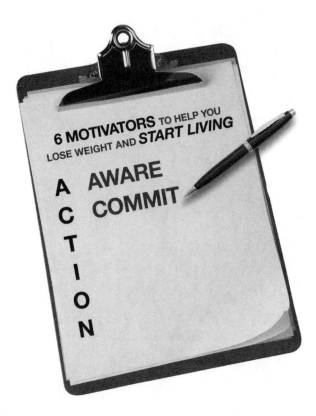

Commit

The next step in your journey toward greater health is to **commit** to living a disciplined life and to winning over temptation. Change is not easy. If you are going to improve your health and wellness, you have to be committed to using the Bible—your new Playbook—to help you develop a strategy that will help you change, reach your new goals, and overcome the temptation that Satan will use against you to keep you from winning.

Chapter 3

You Gotta Play by the Playbook

Do not be wise in your own eyes; fear the LORD and depart from evil.
It will be health to your flesh, and strength to your bones.

PROVERBS 3:7-8

By now you are probably saying to yourself, *All right, you got me. I know I need to do something. I need to get off the couch, and you've convinced me that in this new game I'm playing, I have to play by the rules of the Playbook—the Bible. But how in the world do I get started?*

I hear you! Remember, for I a long time I was just like you, sitting comfortably in that La-Z-Boy recliner. I knew I needed to change, but change is tough. I was embarrassed at what I had become, and I was struggling with the nagging fear of failure. What if I couldn't lose all the weight? What if I lost it and then put it right back on? I didn't want to talk about my newfound realization—my wake-up call—with anybody. In my mind, if nobody knew that I was actively trying to get healthy again and I failed, there would be no harm, no foul.

I never intended to teach or preach on health, start a weight-loss program in my church, or write a book about having a "Bod4God." I just knew that I needed to commit to doing *something*. Instead of being "wise in my own eyes," as our key verses in Proverbs 3:7-8 state, I had to call out to God and change my ways so that I would have health and strength. So I quietly started making changes on my own, just me and my Bible. I already knew that the Bible was the Rule Book for my life, and once I realized it also had a lot to say about my body and my health, I understood it would also give me the nuts and bolts of how I could accomplish my new goal.

I began to think of the Bible as my *new* Playbook. I remember studying my football playbook in college. We would go over and over the plays that we were working on and how we were going to execute them. Who was going to do what? To where would that person run on the field? The playbook was our guide, our lifeline in the game. In it were all the strategies on how we were going to win.

As Elizabeth Merrill of ESPN writes, "In the NFL, the playbook is a sacred hardbound diary of trust. It's an accumulation of decades' worth of knowledge, tweaked and perfected, sectioned off by scribbles and colored tabs. It's the first thing the fresh meat get when preseason workouts start in the spring and the last thing that is pried from a player's sweaty mitts."[1] The Bible had to become my new guide, my lifeline, in this new game I was playing. I knew that if I looked deep enough, it would provide me with all the strategies I would need to succeed in living a healthy lifestyle.

I also knew that I needed help in committing to discipline. Up to this point, I believed that I *was* living a disciplined life. But the realization that I wasn't disciplined in *all* areas of my life hit me like a linebacker. After all, I worked hard every day. In fact, I was often accused of working too hard. I was dedicated to my ministry and my family. But I was completely undisciplined in the area of my health, wellness, eating habits and physical activity and exercise. I had completely ignored this part of my life for way too long. I knew that I needed to change. So I went back to the Bible to find help.

Remember, I'm a pastor, so I've studied the Bible a lot. I went to Bible college and seminary, and I have the degrees to prove it! I was just never in-

Check Up

Big Belly = Big Kids!
According to a study performed by the Mayo Clinic, due to multiple factors, fathers who are overweight significantly increase the risk of their children becoming obese. Researchers found that overweight fathers raise kids in an environment where high calorie food is always available and physical activity is not encouraged. Conversely, they discovered that fathers who control their children's access to high-calorie food and make exercise a family priority are able to favorably impact their children's weight. A further study cited in the *New England Journal of Medicine* reports that parental obesity more than doubles the risk of adult obesity among both obese and non-obese children under the age of 10.[2]

terested in what the Bible had to say about health, food, exercise and things like that. I needed to read it with a different set of eyes and with a different mindset.

The reality is that people do not preach on these types of topics on a regular basis. I mean, have you ever heard your pastor give a sermon on gluttony? Churches are not talking about it. Pastors are not talking about it. Why? Because many of them are preaching on other sins and condemning people while gravy drips from their chin and onto a napkin tucked into their collars. God says a lot about food in the Bible, but we are not eating it!

Lessons from Daniel

I began looking for godly examples on how to live a healthy and productive life. I found that there are 2,930 characters in the Bible, and surely *one* of them could give me some insight into how I was to begin and how I should proceed. I needed a case study—a real person who could show me how it's done. Then it hit me. What better example could I find to show me how to take care of my body than Daniel? I started to read his story found in Daniel 1:8-16, and it suddenly had new meaning for me.

> But Daniel determined that he would not defile himself by eating the king's food or drinking his wine, so he asked the head of the palace staff to exempt him from the royal diet. The head of the palace staff, by God's grace, liked Daniel, but he warned him, "I'm afraid of what my master the king will do. He is the one who assigned this diet and if he sees that you are not as healthy as the rest, he'll have my head!"
>
> But Daniel appealed to a steward who had been assigned by the head of the palace staff to be in charge of Daniel, Hananiah, Mishael, and Azariah: "Try us out for ten days on a simple diet of vegetables and water. Then compare us with the young men who eat from the royal menu. Make your decision on the basis of what you see."
>
> The steward agreed to do it and fed them vegetables and water for ten days. At the end of the ten days they looked better and more robust than all the others who had been eating from the royal menu. So the steward continued to exempt them from the royal menu of food and drink and served them only vegetables (*THE MESSAGE*).

After studying the story in depth, I came to the realization that healthy habits produce a healthy body. If I didn't get a handle on becoming more disciplined and managing my daily habits and routines, I was never going to live a healthy life. Daniel became my model.

Now, some of you may be saying, "Who was Daniel?" Well, he was a young Jewish boy who was captured by Nebuchadnezzar, King of Babylon, when he invaded Jerusalem in 597 BC. Nebuchadnezzar issued an order that the best of the best among the Jewish men were to be brought to the palace to be trained and prepared for service to the king. Daniel taught me how to manage my habits with his response to the difficult situation in which he found himself.

Follow the Bible Play by Play

The first thing I discovered in reading the story of Daniel was that after he was captured and brought to the palace, he was given the food and drink that the king ate and drank, and he was given daily provisions of the king's delicacies. Now, most men would have thought that was great. "I've been captured, but at least I'm getting great food and drink!" The problem was that the food and drink had been offered to idols, and the Bible specifically forbade Daniel to eat or drink it (see Exodus 34:15). The food also likely did not meet the dietary guidelines God had set for His people in Leviticus 11. Even though it was probably the best of the best, by partaking of it Daniel would have broken the rules set in the Bible. Even though he was in a pretty awful situation—having lost his freedom—Daniel decided he was going to obey God and not eat the food. As Proverbs 3:7-8 states, "Fear the LORD and depart from evil . . . it will be health to your flesh."

Determine Your Goals and Write Them Down

The next thing that caught my attention was that Daniel determined what his goal was going to be. Daniel's life and purpose was to glorify God. He obeyed and revered God in all circumstances—even when faced with a buffet.

Let's imagine what Daniel's life at the palace would be like during this time. A signal for the arrival of lunch sounds. Daniel's stomach growls in hunger, but instead of going to the table, he turns and walks away.

"Hey, Daniel, aren't you coming to lunch?" another servant calls to him.

"No, I'll just eat here. I'm just gonna have these vegetables and water."

"What's with you, man? You should see the goodies in there at the king's table. It's loaded, and you can have anything you want. Come on!"

"Thanks, but I'm fine. The food in there has been offered to gods and idols, and I will not eat it. This meal is fine.

"Okay, but you're gonna waste away to nothing."

Daniel smiles and says, "We'll see."

Just as Daniel set a goal and determined to keep it, I knew that if I was going to manage my habits, I would have to set goals and keep them. For me, my first goal was to lose 100 pounds. That goal became my statement of faith in God—my vision for a healthier future. In Mark 11:23, Jesus said, "Say to that mountain, be removed and it shall be removed." Those 100 pounds were the mountain in my life that needed to be removed, and I needed to constantly be reminded of this goal.

The best way to do this is to write it down. There's just something about writing out a goal or a reminder that cements it in your mind. So I wrote out my goal and posted it everywhere so I could keep it in front of me.

Post-It notes are a great way to keep your goals where you can see them. Put them on your mirror where you shave or dry your hair. Put them where you will be looking at your body so you can say, "I want to do something about this!" Make sure you put them in places at work as well, so when those cookies, donuts and candies come out it will remind you of what you are trying to accomplish. And don't forget the refrigerator! Put a note right there in front of you so that when you go to open the door to grab something out of it, you see it. It will help you to remember that what you want more than anything else is to meet this goal.

As Habakkuk 2:2 says, "Then the Lord answered me and said: 'Write the vision and make it plain on tablets, that he may run who reads it.'"

Create a Roadmap to Your Goals

Mike Shanahan, the current coach of the Washington Redskins, once said that "goals are detailed roadmaps to your dreams." For this reason, when you are determining what your goals should be, make sure that they are specific, achievable and measurable. The acrostic these words form, S-A-M, can help you remember how to structure your goals.

- **Specific:** A goal that states, "I want to lose weight," or, "I want to start walking," is not specific. A specific goal would state, "I want to lose 30 pounds by the end of a 12-week period," or, "I want to walk 30 minutes every day." You might also want to set some intermittent goals, such as, "I want to lose five pounds every three weeks," or, "I will walk at a moderate pace for the next four weeks, and then pick up my pace for the next eight weeks."

- **Achievable:** Making goals that are not achievable is a good way to set yourself up for failure and discouragement. For instance, setting a goal of losing 100 pounds in two months is specific, but it's probably not achievable (it took me 18 months to lose 100 pounds). Experts say that a healthy weight-loss goal is about one to two pounds per week for long-term weight loss. Now, if you are like me and weigh 340 pounds when you start out, you might lose five pounds or more in each of the first few weeks, but your weight loss will eventually level out. Likewise, when determining whether an exercise goal is achievable, determining to run in a 10K race five weeks from now is specific, but again, if you are not in shape, it is probably not achievable.

• **Measurable:** A third point to consider is whether your goal is measurable. This is an easy one. Weight loss is measurable—you can step on the scale to see if you are reaching your goal and measure your waistline to see if it is shrinking. When walking, you can use a pedometer to measure your number of steps; when swimming, you can measure your progress by counting laps; and when weight lifting, you can measure the amount of weight you lift.

Just remember SAM and set specific, achievable and measurable goals, and you will be happy with the results you achieve.

Develop a Strategy

After Daniel set the goal to eat only vegetables and drink only water, he developed a strategy for making his goal a reality. He told his manager in the king's palace to give him and the other Hebrew men with him only water and vegetables for 10 days, and then he stuck to his plan no matter what anyone said.

You are probably asking yourself, *Which plan do I choose?* You are going to have to find a plan that works for you—I can't tell you exactly what that plan should be. You've probably already tried plans where someone told you what to eat and what not to eat and how to exercise. Lasted only a few days, didn't it? However, I *am* going to offer you lots of ideas and tips for how to stick to your playbook.

The important thing to remember is that you need to choose a strategy that is best for you. The first thing to do is to talk to God about it. As David wrote, "The steps of a good man are ordered by the LORD, and He delights in his way" (Psalm 37:23). If you don't know what to do, the Bible says you can ask for wisdom (see James 1:5). Talk to others as well. Proverbs 15:22 states, "Without counsel, plans go awry, but in the multitude of counselors they are established." Just don't try to go it alone—you'll fail.

Follow a Schedule

The next thing Daniel did was to commit to a schedule. He determined what he wanted to do, how he was going to do it, when he was going to do it—and then he did it! It's one thing to come up with a plan and another thing completely to follow through and do it right. However, if you are going to change a habit in your life, you have to commit to following a schedule. Repetition and consistency will help train your body to form new habits and crave new things.

Have a Party

Finally, it's important to celebrate when you accomplish and meet your goal. Create your own Super Bowl celebration. Throw a party! You actually took a swig of water! Man, that is unbelievable! Congratulate yourself. Maybe you didn't eat broccoli, but you actually smelled some and bought it. That is awesome! You tasted an apple. Man, way to go. Keep it up. Pretty soon, you will be craving these things.

What you eat in private you wear in public, so as you start meeting your goals, celebrate the fact that you look better. Focus on progress, not perfection. In Philippians 3:13, Paul says he is "forgetting those things which are behind and reaching forward to those things which are ahead." So forget about the past, all those regrets and all those "wish I hads" and "I should haves." They are over! Just keep your eye on the goal. Focus on moving forward.

After looking at Daniel—this incredible guy who was put in a horrible situation and yet kept his focus and came out on top—I knew that I wanted to commit to this same kind of discipline in my life. I wanted to be like Daniel. So I implemented strategies to win in my life. If you want to win, you have to do the same thing. Do you want people to look at you and see a difference? If so, follow the Bible play by play, determine the goal, create a roadmap, develop a strategy, follow a schedule and throw a party when you succeed.

Belief and Behavior Must Come Together

Sometimes, the biggest obstacle in life isn't what we need to do or even how to do it, but resolving to make the change. At the point when I said, "Enough is enough, I'm sick and tired of being sick and tired," I *believed* I needed to change. I knew that I needed to take better care of myself, and I *believed* I could come up with a plan. The hardest part was committing myself to change my behavior.

My belief and my behavior had to come together. It wasn't enough to want to lose 100 pounds; I had to get up and get moving. I had to come to the realization that in order to make my goal a reality, it would require more determination and action than I had ever before displayed. I was going to have to fight the temptation to stay seated in my La-Z-Boy and indulge night after night in a huge bowl of ice cream. Read on, and I will tell you how I overcame the temptation.

David Conn
Says No More Excuses

LOST 70 POUNDS

Before	**After**

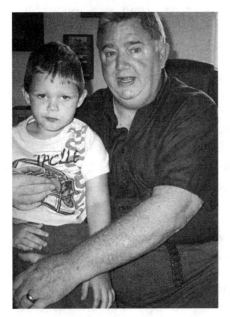 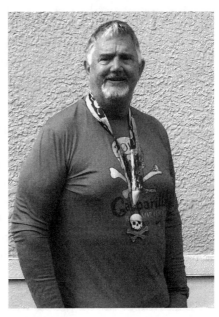

I'm still on my journey, and it has been a long one. I am six-feet, one-inch tall. When I got out of the army, I weighed 185 pounds. Then I gained 30 pounds, which I felt was okay. I still didn't look bad. After I moved to Florida, I started playing tennis, but I didn't lose any weight. My weight would sometimes go up to 260 pounds, and then would go down. I figure I averaged around 245 pounds.

After reading the book *Halftime* by Bob Buford, in which he talks about going from success to significance, I decided to make a job change from real estate to ministry. I had become acquainted with the late Chuck Colson after selling him a house, and he hired me to help with fundraising for Prison Fellowship. I weighed my average—245 pounds—when I went to work for him. One year later, I weighed 270 pounds.

The problem was that when I was fundraising with people of means, they would take me to lunch or dinner. I ate too much and rationalized the reason I did so. I thought, *I can't insult these people by turning down their invitations.* I held the belief that if I was working for God, He would let me slide. Over the next six years, I went from 270 to 320 pounds. That's a weight gain of 50 pounds. The gain was insidious—less than 10 pounds per year—which I didn't think was very much . . . until several years went by.

My doctor used to say, "There's nothing wrong with you, except you're fat." Someone else told me, "There are old people and there are fat people, but there are no old, fat people." I met a wise man named Steve Reynolds, who told me the secret to weight loss is to eat less and exercise more. I dropped 20 pounds in two months, and I thought, *I'll slow down.* Over the course of the next three years I bounced up and down, until I lost a total of 70 pounds.

I decided to run the Gasparella Distance Classic, a half-marathon race held in Tampa Bay, Florida. I entered the race and finished it, which was a big accomplishment. I was exercising more, and I rationalized that because of all the exercise, I could eat more—but I couldn't. I wanted to run, get my weight down another 35 pounds, and not take six years to do it.

The apostle Paul says that your body is the temple of the Holy Spirit. So, if you are losing weight, who are you doing it for? If your body is the temple of the Holy Spirit, you should be treating it as you would a church or temple.

I worked in prisons for 20 years, and the convicts would either ignore or make fun of the fat people who came into the prisons and preached about addictions and having self-control. Just who was the addicted person? Someone once said that the one sin in which you can participate with a pastor is to overeat.

Christians who are reading this book should give their bodies to God as a living sacrifice (see Romans 12:1). Ask God, "Are You happy with what I am doing?" God will show you if He is or not. He is concerned about your witness, and He is also concerned about your physical ability to do what He wants you to do. If you are unhealthy, you may be hindering God's plan in your life.

In Matthew 16:24-25, Jesus says, "If anyone desires to come after Me, let him deny himself, and take up his cross, and follow Me." We are first of all to deny self. That means we can't have everything we want. We can't eat all the chocolate we want and think we are denying our self. When Jesus tells us to pick up our cross, it means there will be things we have to do that we won't want to do. "Deny" stands for "not all the food you want," and your cross will probably be "exercise."

I have two tips for those who want to lose weight to incorporate into their lives. First, you really have to keep a food journal. Statistics prove that those who do lose more weight than those who don't. Second, you need to form a team. I have an email buddy. I need someone to help me stay accountable.

Just remember that a healthy lifestyle is not a destination; it's a journey.

Man Up

Eat Up: Get a Metabolism Boost

Begin the day with breakfast. Research has shown that the people who lose weight and keep it off are the ones who eat breakfast. Choose high fiber foods, such as old-fashioned oatmeal, or whole grain cereals with some fruit. Eating in the morning helps boost your metabolism so you burn more calories. Continue eating four to five mini-meals throughout the day to balance your blood sugar and keep away cravings. You will find by the end of the day that you have actually eaten fewer calories.

Pump Up: Abs for Ads

If you watch TV, trade the "ad" time for some "ab" time. Try holding up a plank. Lie face down, resting on your forearms, with your palms flat on the floor. Push off the floor, raising up onto your toes and then resting on your elbows. Keep your back flat, in a straight line, from head to heels. Tilt your pelvis and contract your abdominals to prevent your rear end from sticking up in the air or your stomach from sagging in the middle. Hold it for the duration of the commercial break.

Reflection and Discussion Questions

1. How is a football playbook like the Bible?

2. What is the strangest food you have ever eaten? What made it strange?

3. What regrets do you have about your current physical condition?

4. In Habakkuk 2:2, the Lord tells the prophet to write the vision He is giving so others can read it. What is the weight-loss goal you have written down? Where will you post it so you will see it throughout your day?

5. It's important to celebrate small successes. What can you celebrate this week? How will you throw a party for this accomplishment?

_____

_____

_____

_____

_____

6. Proverbs 3:7-8 says that when we "fear the Lord" and seek His wisdom for our lives, it will improve our health. What is one big thing you want to do right to follow God's commands and improve your health?

_____

_____

_____

_____

_____

MY PERSONAL GAME PLAN FOR

GETTING IN SHAPE

*Beloved, I pray that you may prosper in all things
and be in health, just as your soul prospers.*

3 JOHN 2

This book is about **ACTION** and about **DOING**! In the spaces below, record what actions you are going to take to improve your health this week.

Aware—I will do the following to show I am aware of my current physical condition and that my body matters to God:

_____
_____
_____
_____
_____

Commit—I will do the following to commit to living a disciplined life and to winning over temptation:

_____
_____
_____
_____
_____
_____

Transform—This is how I will transform the way I think and live:

_____
_____
_____
_____
_____

Incorporate—I will incorporate these healthy eating habits and exercise into my daily life:

_____

_____

_____

_____

_____

Organize—This is how I will organize a team of people to help me win:

_____

_____

_____

_____

_____

Navigate—This is my action plan for healthy living and navigating my way to leaving a lasting legacy:

_____

_____

_____

_____

_____

Chapter 4

Winning Over Temptation

Watch and pray, lest you enter into temptation.
MATTHEW 26:41

"I've lost 25 pounds so far. My biggest problem after I lose the weight is keeping it off. I hope to do better this time around. Lord knows I've lost many pounds in my life many different times. Never has it been permanent."

This was a message I received on Facebook. Sound familiar? It is very common for people who have lost a significant amount of weight to gain it all back. Why does this happen? Well, there could be many reasons to explain a relapse to old habits, but one of the most common is temptation. Get this, guys: Once you have determined to live a disciplined life like Daniel, you had better believe that you will be faced with temptation. It is the clash of the Titans.

A friend told me what it is like on game day in Ann Arbor, Michigan, when the University of Michigan Wolverines play the Ohio State Buckeyes on the gridiron. Locals stay off the streets as thousands of fans pour into the city and take their seats in the famed stadium. Every family with a postage-stamp-sized front lawn turns it into a parking lot. Cops are called in to monitor the traffic and the crowds as these two arch-enemies go head to head. Crowds roar as their team scores, and the cheers can be heard for miles. For each player on the field, it is the battle to end all battles.

Make no mistake: You are in a battle with the devil, and it is a vicious one. Satan wants you to fail. He wants you to destroy yourself with food. He wants you to claim inactivity as your right in life. He is your arch-enemy, and he does not want you to succeed in the game of life.

Satan's Tactics Haven't Changed

Have you ever considered the fact that the first temptation mentioned in the Bible happened in a garden and it involved food? It all started with Adam and Eve and that infamous story about Satan tempting Eve with fruit. Now, I don't know about you, but I can safely say that fruit was never a temptation for me. Ice cream, potato chips and fried chicken maybe, but never an apple or an orange.

Satan was busy trying to destroy people back then, and he is still at it today. He is still using food to tempt people today, just as he did with Eve in the Garden of Eden. Now that you have determined to get up, get moving and start running toward your goal, he will be coming after you stronger than ever. If you are tempted by food, you are going to be tempted by it even more. You have to learn how to tame that temptation and figure out what to do when you want to cheat.

In Genesis 3:6, we read, "When the woman saw that the tree was good for food, that it was pleasant to the eyes, and a tree desirable to make one wise, she took of its fruit and ate. She also gave to her husband with her, and he ate." Why is it that we always want what we can't have? Why do we crave that which is bad for us? Satan understood these desires, and knew exactly what tactics to use on Eve to melt her resistance and cause her to disobey God. In a moment of weakness, she gave up all the amazing benefits of living in the Garden and the closeness of her relationship with God. She gave up life for just one bite of fruit.

When we look at this story, we tend to think poorly of Eve. How could she have disobeyed God? What a fool she was! If only she hadn't been so weak, things would be so different now. But are we any better than Eve? Aren't we guilty of the same kind of weakness and sin every time we eat too much and overindulge in food that is bad for us? Let's face it: we are no better—and no different—than Eve. At our worst, we are trading our lives for momentary pleasures found in food. Satan knows what to put in front of us—what will look good and pleasant to us. He is like the opposing team on the football field, ready to take us out so that we can't score and win the game.

Satan really isn't terribly creative. Like most offenses in football, he has a set number of plays that he keeps using over and over. Satan knows where you are weak, and he will pull just the right play at the right time to fight against your effort to lose weight. He is bent on destroying you. Maybe you will recognize his evil intent, and maybe you won't see it. Maybe you will fall into the trap of believing that giving in to temptation is just a weakness in you.

In football, when teams are faced with an adversary who uses the same tactics frequently, the difference between winning and losing can come down to the coach. When the coach recognizes an opponent is running the same configuration repeatedly, he can shift tactics and direct his offensive to counter the repetitious assault. In your situation, the good news is that you have a Coach who is infallible. He doesn't make mistakes. He sees what Satan is up to, and He can change the way you are playing so you gain the advantage over that old liar. Your Coach is the Holy Spirit, and one of His functions on earth is to help believers overcome the evil one. The Holy Spirit can help you in the grocery store and at the pantry door. He can speak truth into your heart when you pull open the refrigerator door and decide to give up on your plan and eat what you want.

It's time to go on the offensive when it comes to the enemy. In 2 Corinthians 2:11, Paul writes that you "are not ignorant of his devices." Your Coach has told you what he's going to try to put in front of you to stop you so you can be prepared to take him out. When I was playing football, I vividly remember watching films in practice of the guy whom I would be blocking. I would study him over and over the week before the game so I could learn how he operated—where his weaknesses were. I did all of this so that when we met on the field, I would be ready to bring him down. That's the kind of mentality you have to have when it comes to Satan.

We Struggle with the Same Things

Eve's problem was that she wanted something more. She wasn't content with what she had, and she had to have more, no matter what it cost her. The same is true with men today. Just watch the commercials that are played during football games. They are all about Viagra, beer, trucks, girls and having great bodies. The world tells us that in order to be something— to be happy or satisfied—we have to take Viagra, have a beer in our hand, have a nice truck, and have a hot chick at our side. And, just like Eve, many men are taking a bite of the deadly lie that Satan is putting in front of them. But instead of delivering the promised results, it's delivering heartache, addictions, emotional problems and pain.

My weakness was food. That was Satan's target in my life, and it is probably what you are struggling with as well. But there is good news! You *can* beat Satan at his own game. You can overcome and tame temptation by learning to *watch* for his tactics and by strengthening yourself through *prayer*. So write down the key verses at the beginning of every chapter and post them in places where you are likely to be tempted to remind yourself to pray for the Holy Spirit's strength.

Remember that this is your new game, and you are in it to win it! I listened to my Coach and implemented a few strategies into my game plan that have helped me win in my efforts to tame temptation, and hopefully they will do the same for you. Don't let Satan have the upper hand. There is too much at stake. He is seeking to kill and destroy you (see John 10:10), so it's time to suit up, gear up and get ready to take down the opposition.

It's All Around Me—How Do I Handle It?

I admit it: I was an addict! I was addicted to ice cream. From the time I was a child all the way up to 48 years of age, I ate a *huge* bowl of ice cream just about every night. It was my comfort food, my reward after a long hard day's work. After all those years, you had better believe it had become a habit in my life—a very bad habit. So you can imagine how difficult it was for me to stop eating ice cream before I went to bed.

We are all creatures of habit, and our bodies resist change. We also easily revert back to our old ways, even if they are unhealthy. The good news is that as our bodies adapt to new healthy habits, the temptation to cheat will grow less and less over time. Now, I am not saying that this will be easy, because it won't be. It will be hard. But I want to give you hope that you can change and that it is going to get easier and easier.

One of the first things I did when I was starting out was to reward myself with a cheat *meal*. I emphasize the word "meal"—I did not say a cheat "day." I would satisfy a craving I had by telling myself that I would save

Check Up

Big Belly = Feel Depressed
Evidence from the Swedish Obese Subjects Study indicates that obese individuals are three to four times more likely to suffer from clinically significant depression than non-obese individuals. In addition, cases of depression in overweight people are much more serious: depression scores in obese people were as bad or worse than in those with chronic pain. Obesity is linked to other psychological disorders such as eating disorders, distorted body image and low self-esteem. It was found that any physical activity/exercise (even walking) for 30 minutes a day for seven days a week had the equivalent effect to taking a low-dose anti-depressant medication.[1]

this food for my cheat meal, which was usually on Friday night. If I really wanted pizza, I would force myself to stay on track and then reward myself with pizza for that cheat meal.

This was a huge help to me at the beginning. It was my reward after working so hard throughout the week. I had to learn to tell my body what it was going to do and not let it tell me what I was going to do. I also had to trust in the fact that God promises a way of escape for every temptation. As Paul writes in 1 Corinthians 10:13:

> No temptation has overtaken you except such as is common to man; but God is faithful, who will not allow you to be tempted beyond what you are able, but with the temptation will also make a way of escape, that you may be able to bear it.

God promises you a way of escape for every temptation, including food. For me, I've learned to handle temptation by doing three things: (1) pray consistently, (2) shop carefully, and (3) think correctly. I will share more about each of these three things with you right now.

Pray Consistently

You will never overcome temptation without consistent prayer. In Luke 18:1, Jesus said, "Men always ought to pray and not lose heart." God gives you two choices: (1) you can pray and gain strength, which will make you victorious; or (2) you can choose not to pray, which will result in you not having strength and in losing heart. In other words, you can be victorious, or you can fail.

You have to start asking God to help you eat less and exercise more. Just talk to Him and say, "God, please help me. I am no longer looking for that magic potion. I am no longer looking for that diet pill. God, I am willing to face the facts that if I am going to lose weight, I have to eat less and exercise more. And, God, I need Your help to make that happen." Just as you learned in the story of Eve in the Garden, your flesh is weak, but through prayer you can be strong. In Matthew 26:41, Jesus said, "Watch and pray, lest you enter into temptation. The spirit indeed is willing, but the flesh is weak."

In addition to praying that God will help you be strong and overcome temptation, you need to be proactive in praying for your health. I think Christians have it all wrong when it comes to asking God for help in this area. We don't approach prayer for our health from a positive standpoint, but from a negative one.

After pastoring for 30 years, I've learned that when I open up time for prayer requests, about 90 percent of those requests sound like an organ recital. "Oh, this organ is hurting me here, and this organ is hurting me there." "Please pray for this organ, and pray for that organ." Now, if I have a physical problem, I am going to be the first to ask you to pray for me. But I would love to come to a prayer meeting and hear somebody say, "Man, I know I should be drinking more water. Would you all pray that I would do that?" That's the positive-action kind of prayer we should be praying. "Lord, help me get off the couch and start walking," or, "Lord, please help me to overcome the temptation to hit the drive-thru at McDonald's."

Guys, let's face it. We tend to want to do things by ourselves. We like to go solo and do things our own way. We hate asking for directions! But when it comes to temptation, we have to realize that we can't overcome it on our own and through our own strength. We need God to help us. So start praying about what is tempting you and causing you to cheat.

Shop Carefully

The next thing you have to do is to shop carefully. I found my motivation in this area in Romans 13:14, where Paul says, "Put on the Lord Jesus Christ, and make no provision for the flesh, to fulfill its lusts." You have to understand that the battleground is not your kitchen—the battleground is at the *store*.

If you are going to overcome the temptation to cheat, you have to begin dealing with the problem at the grocery store, because if food gets *near* you, it is eventually going to get *in* you. You have to shop for your health, not your happiness, and keep unhealthy foods out of your grocery basket. If you do so, you will keep these foods out of your car. And if you keep them out of your car, you can keep them out of your kitchen. And if you keep them out of your kitchen, you can keep them out of your stomach.

Sounds simple, right? But if you lose the battle at the grocery store, you will soon find yourself praying, "Oh, Lord, help me. Here I am, Lord. I mean, Lord, those potato chips are up in the cupboard—but, Lord, I know that You are going to give me the strength not to touch them. Oh, Lord, please help me."

Whoa, man! The time you should be praying for the strength to overcome the temptation of those potato chips is when you are in aisle number 12. You should find yourself praying, "Lord, this cart is trying to go down aisle number 12. But, Lord, I want to keep it in the aisles where the healthy food is located. So help me keep moving and not go down that aisle."

So, in a nutshell, what does it mean to shop carefully? First, make sure you have eaten before you go into the store so you aren't hungry while shopping. When you are hungry, everything looks good. Second, pray for the infilling of the Holy Spirit as you walk into the store so you won't fulfill the lusts of the flesh. Third, make sure you shop the *outside* of the store. Why? Because the living food—the good stuff that God made, like fruits and vegetables—are located on the outside of the store. Living food will start to die in a few days and must be replaced, so store personnel need to keep it close to the perimeter so they have better access to replenish and replace it. The more you shop on the outside of the store, the healthier you are going to be. The more you shop up and down the aisles, the less healthy you will be.

Finally, read all of the food nutrition labels. I don't buy anything without reading the label. You need to know what you are purchasing and what is in the food that you are about to purchase. By the way, the best foods do not even have a label. Some have a code sticker, and that's all. Finishing your shopping by finding some snacks that are healthy, and have those available when you get hungry.

Think Correctly

The third step in overcoming temptation is to think correctly. In 2 Corinthians 10:5, Paul says that we must cast down "arguments and every high thing that exalts itself against the knowledge of God" and bring "every thought into captivity to the obedience of Christ." We have to understand that every sin begins in the mind. Think about sexual sin. Where does it start? In fact, the biggest sex organ you have in your body is your brain! Every sexual sin starts in the mind.

We have disobedient thoughts not only about sex and other obsessive sins but also about food. We get thoughts of food in our mind and start craving things. But Paul says that we have to cast those disobedient thoughts down. We have to learn to bring "every thought into captivity to the obedience of Christ." We have to take those thoughts that are calling to us to eat this and eat that. We have to take captive those thoughts that tell us, *I don't want to go exercise. I am too tired tonight. I can do it another time.* We have to focus on the fact that short-term pleasure is not worth long-term pain. Yes, this thing that we're being tempted with might be nice in the short term, but what is it going to do to us in the long term? How will we feel in an hour? In two hours?

Sin is fun. Yes, you heard me right. Don't let anybody tell you that sin isn't fun. Actually, sin is a blast! And remember, gluttony is a sin. But it's only fun for a season, and then there is great sorrow. Just think back to the story of Eve. That fruit probably tasted amazing, but the taste of it likely became bitter after she realized the consequences of her one moment of weakness.

I Messed Up—Now What?

Remember, we are all human, and because of that one fateful day in the Garden of Eden, we all deal with our flesh—our sin nature. There is no getting around it. We are going to fail at some point in the game. Even the best teams and players make mistakes. How many times have you been watching a game on TV and your favorite player has blown it and made a crucial error? You probably got all riled up and started yelling at him through the TV, as if he could hear you. It's easy to criticize the refs and the coaches and lose sight of just how hard it is down there on the field.

You and I *will* fail at times. But you have to remember that failure is not final! When you stumble, you need to pick yourself up, move forward, and learn from it. When I cheat, I always think, *How did I get myself in this situation? How can I avoid this situation in the future?* When you fail, you have to say to yourself, *Don't look back—get back on track!*

Proverbs 24:16 says that "a righteous man may fall seven times and rise again." He will what!? That's right, each time he falls he will rise back up again, and that's exactly what you need to do when you fail. Rise up again and keep at it. I've learned over the years that 90 percent of life is showing up.

So determine that you are going to get back up when you fall and that you are going stay in the game. Don't let Satan keep you down. Don't quit, because if you keep on with your *commitment* to live a healthy lifestyle, before you know it, a *transformation* will take place in your life, your attitudes, your desires and your body!

Alvie Tosh
Beats the Big Mac Attack

LOST 63 POUNDS

Before	After
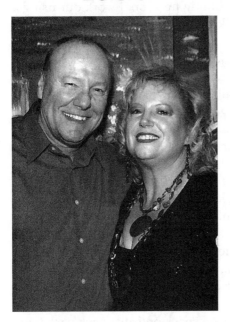	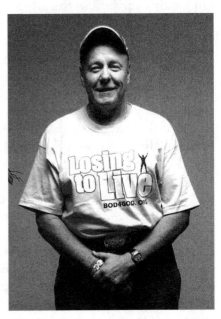

I was a yo-yo dieter until my wife and I heard about the Losing to Live weight-loss competition. We had always wanted to change, but we had been unable to do so, even with all the diets we had tried. My wife and I were both exhausted, and the doctors wanted to give us medicine. So we decided that since we had tried everything else, there might be something to be said for including God.

We checked into the program and decided to try it. The first night I listened to everything that was being said and found it interesting, but I wasn't sure if it was for me. I went to the class and again I found it interesting, but I still didn't know if it was for me. I was still skeptical during the second class. However, I am very competitive, and when we started the competition, I wondered if I could do it. I decided to try. The first week, I *gained* a pound. I have to confess that my heart wasn't in it.

Then I started hearing the stories of others in the group, and I realized that most were losing. I wasn't. There was one lady in our class who hadn't lost anything, so I made up my mind to lose a pound for her as a way to show my support. After that second week, I lost six pounds.

I feel accountable to my team. I don't want to let them down, and I don't want to let myself down either. I enjoy the program, I feel better, and I'm looking forward to the 5K race coming up soon. I work out using a treadmill and exercise bike, and I walk the dog while wearing a 40-pound weight vest.

A recent situation has shown me just how much I have changed. I am what you would call an "emotional eater," and I grew up eating Southern food. (When that type of food is all you know, you eat it—until you decide to change.) A couple of weeks ago, something emotional happened to me, and I wanted to eat a Big Mac. Then I thought about it, and decided I really didn't want the Big Mac after all. It was then that I realized I *have* changed.

At the beginning of the Losing to Live competition, I set a goal of weighing 200 pounds. Today, I have lost 63 pounds. I went from size 40 pants to a size 34. At one time I wouldn't look in the mirror, but now I look and think, *Not too bad.*

To accomplish my weight loss and become healthier, I had to change my eating habits. I started eating more fruit and vegetables. (In fact, I've eaten more fruit during the competition than I ever had before.) I mix up tuna fish with fat-free mayo and relish and eat it right out of the bowl, or sometimes I put it on bread or crackers. I snack on fruit snack packs.

I feel guilty if I eat the wrong foods, so now I don't eat them. I haven't had a candy bar in I don't know how long. It took about two weeks for me to get over sugar and salt cravings, but eating healthy has been worth it. Now my exhaustion is gone, and it feels as if I am eating the right foods all day long. I am so thankful that my wife is helping me. We both cook, which keeps us on track. On Saturday mornings, we weigh in and then go out for breakfast. It's a kind of cheat meal, but it helps us to stay on track the rest of the week.

One other thing I enjoy doing is playing softball with our church team. Exercise is important, and I've taken this for my motto: "Eat every day you exercise." My weight loss has added to my confidence level and physical ability. At one time I couldn't reach down to pick up a softball. Now I can. I know I'm on the right track.

If you are discouraged, don't give up. Find someone to encourage you. Get an email buddy to help you through the tough days. And have faith. I know I don't want to go back to what I was, and you won't want to either once you get on track. It's worth all it takes to get healthy.

Man Up

Eat Up: How to Eat a Rainbow

Conquer cravings by "eating the rainbow." Fill your plate each day with different colors of fruits and vegetables to give your body a boatload of nutrients that will fill you up, give you more energy, and keep you satisfied. When you put high-quality fuel in your body, it feels so good, and it helps you not to be as susceptible to temptation. When you fill up on vegetables, you will be gaining health *and* cutting calories.

Pump Up: Compress Your Stress

Keep a foam-compression ball at your desk and squeeze it throughout the day. This will work the muscles in your wrists, forearms and fingers and improve your overall grip strength. Start by doing a one-minute round, and then switch hands and repeat. Remember, a strong man has strong hands.

Reflection and Discussion Questions

1. In what ways is your battle against weight a direct attack by Satan?

2. What is your greatest food temptation?

3. What do you tell yourself when you don't want to exercise?

4. To overcome temptation, you must pray consistently, shop carefully, and think correctly. Of these three, which is your greatest weakness? What can you do to improve in that area?

5. How do you respond when you mess up? What would you like to change about the way you respond?

_____

_____

_____

_____

_____

6. In Matthew 26:41, Jesus says we need to "watch" for temptation. What are three things you need to watch out for to be more healthy?

_____

_____

_____

_____

_____

MY PERSONAL GAME PLAN FOR

GETTING IN SHAPE

Beloved, I pray that you may prosper in all things
and be in health, just as your soul prospers.
3 JOHN 2

This book is about **ACTION** and about **DOING**! In the spaces below, record what actions you are going to take to improve your health this week.

Aware—I will do the following to show I am aware of my current physical condition and that my body matters to God:

_____
_____
_____
_____
_____

Commit—I will do the following to commit to living a disciplined life and to winning over temptation:

_____
_____
_____
_____
_____

Transform—This is how I will transform the way I think and live:

_____
_____
_____
_____
_____

Incorporate—I will incorporate these healthy eating habits and exercise into my daily life:

_____

_____

_____

_____

_____

Organize—This is how I will organize a team of people to help me win:

_____

_____

_____

_____

_____

Navigate—This is my action plan for healthy living and navigating my way to leaving a lasting legacy:

_____

_____

_____

_____

_____

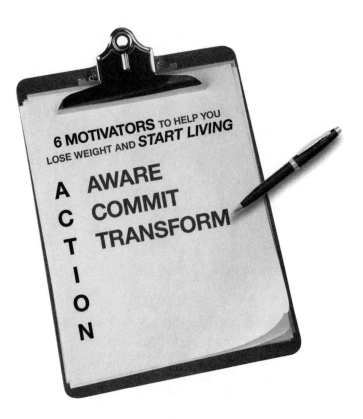

Transform

The third step in your journey toward greater health is to **transform** the way you think and the way you live. Your thought life will make or break you. It's time to stop listening to Satan, the father of foul play, and start meditating on the truth found in God's Word. Once you transform your thinking, it's time to start transforming your doing. Stop making excuses and start producing positive change in your life.

Chapter 5

Get Your Head in the Game

For those who live according to the flesh set their minds on the things of the flesh, but those who live according to the Spirit, the things of the Spirit.
ROMANS 8:5

"Setting a goal is not the main thing," former Dallas Cowboys head coach Tom Landry told his players, "it is deciding how you will go about achieving it and staying with that plan."

I love this quote! It says that *what you think is what you do*. In the words of Paul in Romans 8:5, if we set our minds on things of the flesh, what we will get is a fleshly life—and for some of us, it's too much flesh. All joking aside, this is a powerful principle to understand. Your thought life is vitally important and is a key component in winning at anything in life. You can make all kinds of great plans and set wonderful goals, but if you aren't determined to implement a plan to achieve them, all of those best-laid plans will amount to nothing.

So, now that you are *aware* you need to make a change to your physical condition and lifestyle, and now that you know nothing will change until you *commit* to change, it's time to figure out how to *transform* your thinking to change your life.

Football isn't just a physical game; it's also a mental game. It isn't enough to have strength and skill; you also have to have the mindset and strategy to win. Coaches spend a lot of time mentally preparing their players to win by showing them how to read the players on the opposing team, anticipate plays, and constantly change their strategy based on how the game is being played. Team members must stay focused on what their job is as a team member, for if players fail to focus, they could cost the team the game. Players can't afford to let themselves get distracted and lose sight of the goal.

These same principles apply to us as well. Before we can start focusing on the physical side of the game of getting healthy, we have to get our minds focused. We have to get our head in the game, and we have to transform our thinking. Like Coach Landry said, we have to set goals for ourselves and then determine to stick to a plan so we can meet those goals.

We all want to win big and have success at what we do. The cool thing is that if we have the right thinking—the right mindset—we can win big. We just have to train our minds to think about the right things. This takes work, and for a lot of us it means performing a complete overhaul of our thought life. We have to change how we feel about our bodies, how we feel about health, how we feel about food and exercise, and how we feel about our future. We may even have to change how we feel about our past.

Dealing with these feelings and emotions is going to be hard—necessary, but hard. After all, these thoughts and feelings have taken root in our minds, and it is only through careful and deliberate execution that we will be able to shift our thinking in the right direction. Think of it as exercise for your mind. You have to train your mind to believe that you are valuable to the Creator instead of worthless junk. You have to train your mind to think differently about food and exercise. You have to exercise your thought life to focus on living a healthy and productive life.

How Do I Change My Mind?

Now, I know many of you are asking yourself, *I know that I don't want to think as I always have, but how do I think differently? How do I change my mind?* Take a look at what Paul says in Romans 12:1-2:

> I beseech you therefore, brethren, by the mercies of God, that you present your bodies a living sacrifice, holy, acceptable to God, which is your reasonable service. And do not be conformed to this world, but be transformed by the renewing of your mind, that you may prove what is that good and acceptable and perfect will of God.

In this passage, God tells us how to change our mindset: Don't conform; be transformed! In other words, we are not to think as the world thinks. The world wants us to believe that we can do whatever we want with our bodies. We can drink whatever we want, eat whatever we want, live however we want. It's the eat-drink-and-be-merry type of thinking. But this is contrary to what the Bible says about the way in which we should live.

We have already examined how the Bible says we were made by God and for God and that our bodies are not our own. Our bodies are to be holy, living sacrifices that we present to God. So, the first step in changing our mind is not to *conform* our thinking to the world. The next step is to be *transformed,* and the first thing we must understand is that we can't transform ourselves. The only way we can change our thinking or "renew our minds" is with God's guidance. He does the transforming through His Word, the Bible, and as we read the Word and meditate on the Creator's plans for our bodies and our lives, He will begin to change how we think.

We are constantly being bombarded by messages from the world as to what is a good and acceptable game plan for our life. Satan is at work in this world, and he uses these lying messages to keep us in bondage to our sin and destruction. However, the more we line ourselves up with the Word of God, the more His truth will be revealed to us, and the more our thought life will naturally fall into line with His plan for our lives. If we don't transform our thinking, and if we continue to listen to the lies that Satan subtly whispers in our ears, we will continue on a downward spiral that leads to death.

When we commit to reforming our worldly thinking and mindsets, and when we constantly renew our minds and transform our thinking by reading God's Word, we will change the way we think. At this point, we will begin to really see positive change and success. Our thought life is our most powerful tool in this game we are playing. It will determine if we win or lose. If we let negative thinking and doubt control what we do, we won't achieve our goals. But if we think on things that are positive and are true, we will start winning.

The Power of Thought

Johnny Curtis, a mixed martial arts trainer and professional fighter, teaches his fighters the importance of focusing their thoughts and dealing with the doubts that come to all competitors—even though they have trained hard and know what to do. Curtis's background is in wrestling. He was a two-time All-American wrestler and a member of the United States national team.[1]

Curtis believes that fighters need to figure out what their main weapons are. "For the men I train, focusing starts a few weeks out from a fight," he says. "I'm big on having a game plan—something the men can focus on as the fight draws near. Suppose a wrestler is fighting a boxer. The wrestler can't just stand there; he'll get smashed in the face. He needs to think through his skills and his moves, decide where he is the strongest, and figure ways to get the boxer to 'bend' to his game."

Curtis finds that men don't like to spend time working on their weaknesses due to fear that they will fail or look stupid. He tells them, "If you're going to fail, fail forward. Fear of failure will limit an athlete's success. It will also limit weight-loss success or exercise success or any other kind of success there is. In Proverbs 26:13, we read, 'The lazy man says, "There is a lion in the road!"' It's an excuse that the scared man uses as well."

Curtis goes on to say, "Many athletes train the body but do not focus enough on training the mind. This is where a game plan comes in. You think through how you will deal with your opponent. You play it out in

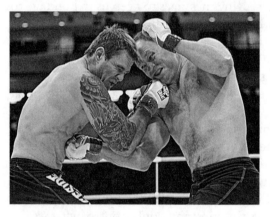

your head over and over. You ask, 'How do I see myself attacking him?' A match is made up of three parts: pre-competition, competition and post competition. The 'pre' part includes having a game plan with measurable goals embedded in it, learning the game plan, running the plays again and again until they are automatic, and conditioning the body. For some wrestlers, all the training goes out the window when they start the actual competition. They just jump in and start wrestling without a plan."

For Curtis, the nerves really kick in about a week before the competition. While he acknowledges it's normal to feel anxious when looking forward to a competition, he finds it is at this time that self-doubt, discouragement and other negative emotions come flying at him. He states, "We need to take heed to what Martin Luther said: 'We can't control the birds that fly over our head, but we don't have to let them land on our head and make a nest in our hair.'"

Curtis notes that Satan likes to shoot his fiery darts at our minds, and when those negative thoughts come our way, we need to resist the devil and he will flee from us (see James 4:7). We have to replace those negative thoughts with positive ones. As he has learned, "When the fight day gets closer, we will be tempted to anticipate every conceivable problem that could come up. But we must not do that! Past failures have to be tossed out. We can't expect to feel 100 percent on the day of competition. We have to disregard the fact that we feel only about 85 percent ready and not waste time focusing on stuff we can't control. We can't create our own stress. If we have trained faithfully, we are ready, and it is never helpful to focus on how we feel. So what if we had a bad week of practice! Forget it. It doesn't help to keep all this negative-thinking junk between our ears. We have to replace it with positive thoughts."

Curtis states that unpleasant things will happen in every competition that will be out of our control—things like a horrible call from a referee that breaks our concentration and takes us mentally out of the game, or a wrong play that causes us to lose our concentration—we must refuse to melt down and remain fully committed to getting the job done. "I see my sport like a physical chess match," he says. "There is a strategy the opponent is playing. I have an idea about my opponent's game, and my opponent has an idea about mine. I'm trying to figure out how to win, and I'm totally committed to the game and to winning. A partial commitment is no commitment."

Something that helps Curtis overcome negative thinking is to have Scripture tucked into his head that he can pull out in weak moments. One such passage is Philippians 4:6-9, in which Paul—who wrote these words while under house arrest in Rome—tells us exactly how to overcome negative thinking:

Be anxious for nothing, but in everything by prayer and supplication, with thanksgiving, let your requests be made known to God; and the peace of God, which surpasses all understanding, will guard your hearts and minds through Christ Jesus. Finally, brethren, whatever things are true, whatever things are noble, whatever things are just, whatever things are pure, whatever things are lovely, whatever things are of good report, if there is any virtue and if there is anything praiseworthy—meditate on these things. The things which you learned and received and heard and saw in me, these do, and the God of peace will be with you.

"Paul is telling us to forget about our circumstances, excuses, aches and pains and think on the good," Curtis says. "He is telling us to focus on the positive. We are the only ones who can control the thoughts we allow to camp out between our ears—and it *is* possible for all of us to control those thoughts. So let me encourage you to stand up, be a man, and get the job done. If you are injured, that's a short-term deal. Obesity, on the other hand, is a big deal—a life-threatening big deal. It's time to stop the denial, stop the fear, stop the excuses and get real about weight loss and exercise."

The Father of Offensive Foul Play

We can't talk about the battle that takes place in our minds without talking a bit more about the fiercest opponent we will ever face: Satan. As we have discussed, he is lying in wait to tempt you in any way he can. He wants to knock you down and keep you there by distorting the truth and playing tricks with your mind. He has carefully crafted several offensive lies to keep you there on the couch—to keep you from making progress down the field of life and reaching your goal.

As Jesus says in John 8:44, Satan was "a murderer from the beginning, and does not stand in the truth, because there is no truth in him. When he speaks a lie, he speaks from his own resources, for he is a liar and the father of it." You are his target, and he wants to destroy you. The sad fact is that if you are slowly killing yourself with a knife, a fork and an ice cream spoon, you are helping Satan accomplish his mission—you are doing his dirty work for him. This is why *you have to stop*. You have to recognize the lies that he is using to keep you from getting healthy and strong.

Check Up

Big Belly = High Cost

Studies by the Centers for Disease Control (CDC) have shown that obesity and overweight have a significant impact on the U.S. healthcare system, through both direct and indirect costs. Direct costs include the amounts spent on actual patient care, whereas the indirect costs include factors such as decreased productivity, absenteeism and days of missed work. Combined, the CDC calculated that in 2008 obesity and overweight cost more than $147 billion. A subsequent study conducted by the Cornell University department of economics in 2012 showed that even those numbers did not adequately represent the problem—they calculated that obese and overweight individuals cost, on average, $2,741 per year more in healthcare cots than non-overweight individuals, for a total of more than $190 billion. The Cornell study estimated that up to 21 percent of U.S. healthcare spending is on overweight and obese individuals. Furthermore, in 2007–2008 (at the height of the U.S.'s conflicts in Iraq and Afghanistan), 1 in 4 applicants to the U.S. armed services were denied entry due to being overweight or obese. Obesity is the leading cause for disqualification for military recruits, which suggests that obesity affects our national security.[2]

In the next few pages, we are going to get to the heart of Satan's deception. We are going to look at seven deadly lies that Satan is either using right now or is going to use against you. It's time to be honest with yourself and take responsibility for your past actions and your way of thinking. This isn't going to be easy, but it will be worth it in the end.

Satan's Seven Deadly Lies

Lie #1 — Failure: You're Not Going to Succeed

Have you ever found yourself saying, "I've tried everything to lose weight in the past, but no matter what I try it just doesn't work for me"? Or how about, "I just blew my diet for this week, so perhaps I'll have better luck if I try next week"? If so, these are lies that Satan is using against you to keep you focused on your past failures and prevent you from moving forward. He is whispering, "Why try? You are just going to fail." He wants to keep you in bondage and stuck in the mentality that you can't do it.

Don't fall prey to this lie and get discouraged. Don't focus on the past. Quit looking in the rearview mirror of your life. Keep your focus and attention on the future and on Paul's words in Philippians 4:13: "I can do all things through Christ who strengthens me."

Maybe you haven't succeeded in the past because you have been going about it in the wrong way. You have to keep in mind that it takes more than willpower to gain long-term success. When it comes to improving your health, a diet isn't going to bring about long-term change—it's going to take developing a healthy lifestyle plan built around eating less and exercising more. And you can't do it halfway. You have to be sold out for change. You have to be determined, and you have to create a sustainable plan of action.

Once you come up with your plan, you also have to stick with it. In Luke 14:28-30, Jesus says, "Which of you, intending to build a tower, does not sit down first and count the cost, whether he has enough to finish it—lest, after he has laid the foundation, and is not able to finish, all who see it begin to mock him, saying, 'This man began to build and was not able to finish'?" Quit allowing Satan to tackle you and make you think you are going to fail. If you create a healthy lifestyle plan built around the principles found in God's Word and stick to it, you can't fail!

Lie #2 — Time: You Don't Have Time to Lead a Healthy Life

This is a lie I hear a lot. "I just don't have the time." "I'm too busy to exercise." "I don't even have time to eat lunch as it is, much less take extra time for breakfast." And then there's the shopping for and preparing healthy meals excuse. My favorite one is this: "I'm really busy right now, but I'll start tomorrow." It's the mañana diet mentality. Then tomorrow turns into next week . . . and then next month . . . and then after the holidays. Satan loves to use the time clock against you. If he can get you to believe you are too busy to fit healthy or spiritual things into your life, he can succeed at keeping you in bondage. He wants to steal every minute so you won't use your minutes for activities that glorify God.

Let's face it; we are all busy people. As a pastor of a growing church, nobody was busier than I was. But I had to come to grips with the fact that Satan was lying to me—and that I had believed his lie. Remember that your body was made by God and for God, and you have to be a manager of that wonderful body God created. This means making the time to care for it. In Ephesians 5:15-16, Paul says, "See then that you walk circumspectly, not as fools but as wise, redeeming the time, because the days are evil." You only have one body, so don't waste it! Yes, it does take time each day to care for it, but if you don't invest that time, you are headed for big health issues.

Think of the way you take care of your car. Do you say to yourself, *Oh, I don't have time to get an oil change. I'll just keep driving it until it breaks down.* Of course not! That would be crazy. It's common knowledge that changing the oil in your car will keep it running better and for a longer period of time. The same is true of your body. If you are taking care of it in the way you should, you are going to feel better and be able to do more for a longer period of time.

When you say to yourself, *I'll start tomorrow,* you are using the procrastination excuse. The truth is that most of the time the "I'll start tomorrow" part never comes—and if you don't start losing weight and getting healthy, you are guaranteed to have fewer tomorrows. So don't believe the lie that you don't have time to get healthy. If you don't start making time to do this, you may not have much time left!

Lie #3—Fear: You Might Hurt Yourself (or Even Die!)

I've actually had people tell me that they have heard stories of thin, healthy people keeling over dead from running or exercising too much. Satan loves to use these types of fear tactics on you. He knows that if he can get you to believe that exercising might be harmful to your health, you will stay on the couch.

For this reason, before beginning a new eating and exercising regimen, make an appointment with a doctor to get expert advice on what your body can handle and how you should begin. Your doctor may need to do certain tests to make sure your body can handle the increased exercise level. If you have had a heart attack or stroke, your doctor may put limits on your maximum heart rate or require you to monitor your blood pressure. Regardless, I'm certain that your doctor will want you to *move*. In fact, your doctor will probably encourage you to start moving.

Remember, you are fearfully and wonderfully made (see Psalm 139:14). God created your body to move! Fear of hurting yourself is just an excuse and a lie that Satan will use to keep you from getting healthy. So when these fears strike, listen to God's words in Joshua 1:9: "Have I not commanded you? Be strong and of good courage; do not be afraid, nor be dismayed, for the LORD your God is with you wherever you go." Did you hear that? "The LORD your God is with you wherever you go." Don't be afraid!

Lie #4—Denial: You Don't *Really* Have a Problem

"Don't worry about me. I don't have a problem. After all, I'm not as heavy as so-and-so. You need to be talking to him about his weight. Anyway, my few extra pounds aren't hurting anyone but me. It is nobody's business. I wish people would just let me be."

Sound familiar? Satan will use these thoughts to keep you from facing your sin and your faults. He wants to keep you in denial so you never move on to bigger and better things. He wants to keep your attention focused on those around you instead of on God and what He wants for your life.

God doesn't grade on a curve! You are accountable for your actions, and you need to take your eyes off others and start focusing on your own health. Sure, you will always be able to find people who are worse off than you are. But, just like you, they will have to give an account as to how they have lived their lives. In Romans 14:4, Paul says, "Who are you to judge another's servant? To his own master he stands or falls. Indeed, he will be made to stand, for God is able to make him stand."

It's time to take responsibility for your own actions and to admit that you do have a problem. It's the only way to move forward.

Lie #5—Blame: It's Not Your Fault

None of us like to admit that we are to blame. In fact, blame-shifting seems to be a way of life today. A lot of stories I hear from people start with these words: "You don't understand . . . there's a reason why I'm so heavy. I have issues." I am sure you have experienced circumstances in your life that are difficult to bear, but I have to say it: *Quit feeling sorry for yourself!* You have been listening to Satan's and the world's psychobabble for too long. It is time to break Satan's hold and move into victory.

In 2 Corinthians 1:3-4, Paul says, "Blessed be the God and Father of our Lord Jesus Christ, the Father of mercies and God of all comfort, who comforts us in all our tribulation." You must stop seeking your comfort in food and instead seek comfort in the God of all comfort. God created food to be fuel for your body, not therapy for how you feel. Food cannot heal your broken heart, make your children listen to you, stop your spouse from nagging you, or fill a void in your life. Only God can do these things. He knows you better than anyone else because He created you. He knows what you are going through. Your obesity is only adding another issue to your life, and you need to deal with it. So quit shifting the blame to someone or something else! Take ownership of your actions, seek wise counsel, and for comfort look to the loving God who created you.

Lie #6—Difficulty: It's too Hard for You

"I just cannot do it. When I exercise I get winded, and my lungs feel as if they are on fire. My muscles get sore. I get lightheaded. It is just such hard work. The next morning I'm stiff and can hardly get out of bed. I feel like I'm going to die. It is easier to just keep living as I have rather than put myself through all of this discomfort."

Can you relate to these statements? Satan wants you to believe that you can't lead a healthy lifestyle. It is true that exercising is going to be difficult at first, but Satan is using half-truths to confuse you. It is *hard*, but it's not *too hard*. It's not impossible. It's not called a "workout" for nothing. You will be *working*.

Fight this lie by refusing to believe that everything must always be comfortable and convenient. Stop being lazy and start focusing on becoming the healthy man God created you to be. Don't be like the sluggard described in Proverbs 26:15, who "buries his hand in the bowl; it wearies him to bring it back to his mouth." It's time to stop focusing on how difficult it is to get healthy and just do it.

Lie #7—Emotions: You Won't Feel Better About Yourself

This lie starts off like this: "I just don't feel like eating right or exercising." I've heard people use excuses such as, "I don't feel good," or, "I'm too tired." People who have bought into this lie do not believe that eating right and exercising will improve their quality of life and how they feel.

Satan wants you to focus on yourself and the here-and-now. He wants you to focus on how you feel in the moment and not how much better you will feel in the long run. It's like the example of the car in need of work that we discussed in Lie #2. If you never change the oil and ignore the preventative maintenance, your car may run fine for a while, but eventually it's going to shut down. In the same way, you can ignore the preventative maintenance you need to do on your body for a season, but eventually you will feel the serious consequences of your actions.

It is important to understand that you cannot base your decisions in life on *feelings;* you have to base them on *facts.* The fact is that if you don't take care of your body—if you don't deal with the issues of your health right now—you will pay later. Sure, you don't feel like getting moving and changing your eating habits, but the fact is that the decision to do so will reap many positive results later.

The good news is that when you do get up off the couch, you will start feeling better than you have in years. Whenever I don't feel like going to the gym, I think about Paul's words in 1 Corinthians 9:27: "But I discipline my body and bring it into subjection, lest, when I have preached to others, I myself should become disqualified." I want to live a disciplined life and healthy life so I can lead others and be an encouragement to them. To do this, I have to stop focusing on how I feel!

Listen to the Coach

There you have it, guys—the seven deadly lies that Satan will try to use on you again and again. Remember that he isn't very creative and that he isn't dreaming up new ways to attack you. He doesn't have to do so, because he can get people to keep falling for the same dumb plays over and over. It's time to stop listening to him.

Whenever you feel Satan beside you whispering one of his lies into your ear, become that little boy who sticks his fingers in his ears and says, "La-la-la-la-la-la-la. . . . I can't hear you!" Tune Satan out and listen to your new Coach, God. Remember, God wants to speak truth into your life every day through the pages of His Word. He wants you to live, and He wants you healthy.

Meditate on the Scriptures in each section above. Memorize as many as you can so that when the enemy starts to throw doubt your way, you have a ready defense. Learn to focus your thinking and not be distracted. Your Coach wants you to win, and once you get your head in the game and start thinking like a winner, you can start working your way toward the goal, play by play and yard by yard, until you reach the end zone. You can't win until you get in the game, so focus on progress, not perfection. We will talk more about that subject in the next chapter.

Israel Villanueva
Cries Out for Heavenly Help

LOST 30 POUNDS

Before	After
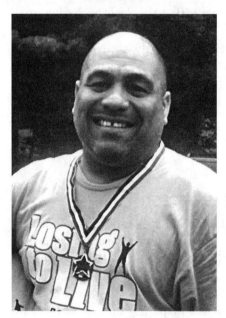	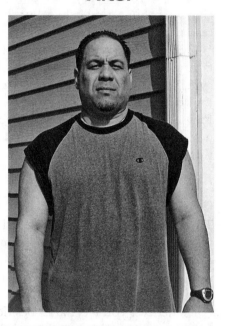

I got up to 260 pounds after I left the Army, and it was a real wake-up call for me when the doctor told me I needed to exercise. My wife and I got down on our knees in our living room and started praying and asking God to help us. A few months later we came to Capital Baptist Church and heard Pastor Steve preach a series on Losing to Live. People in the congregation had seen that he had lost weight, and they wanted to know what he was doing. So he told them in that series.

Pastor Steve inspired us, and we started meeting as a group and talking about having a weight-loss competition. It was the answer to the prayer my wife and I had cried out to God in our living room. I lost 30 pounds, but then I pulled a muscle and had to lay off exercise for two months. I started gaining weight again. My wife wanted to try a program our doctor recommend called Medifast, and he said that he would monitor our progress on it. I just knew that whatever we did, I needed to stay with Losing to Live as my base. When *Bod4God: The Four Keys to Weight Loss* came out, I read it, and it really made sense to me. My wife and I formed our own support group.

A diet is not lifestyle change. True change only comes through dedication, inspiration, eating correctly, exercising and becoming part of a team. I have taken Revelation 4:11 as my theme verse: "You are worthy, O Lord, to receive glory and honor and power; for You created all things, and by Your will they exist and were created." I have that verse on my desk, and I look at it every day. It reminds me that I am here to please God, and I want God to be pleased with me in all areas of my life.

Today, I take the *Bod4God* CDs to the gym. They are about 30 to 40 minutes long, so if I exercise for that length of time, it provides a good workout. I prefer to use the elliptical machine, and I try to burn 20 calories per minute. I challenge myself so I don't get bored. At the end of my workout, I walk slowly on the treadmill for 30 minutes to cool down. I walk until my heart rate is in the 90s, and then I stop. I bought a watch that measures my heart rate and calories burned so I can know at all times how I am doing. My father once told me that the heart is like an old-fashioned pressure cooker. You have to control the pressure on the cooker or it will blow. I know that having too much pressure on my heart will cause it to blow, so I want to exercise and stay healthy.

I strongly believe that I needed God's help to lose weight. Everything began with Him. I was so desperate and scared when the doctor warned me of the seriousness of my condition, and I needed to change. I know that on my own, I will fail, but when I depend on God and look for ways to please Him, I will succeed.

I want to be around for my son and daughter when they get married. I want to influence my grandchildren. I know you do too. We are all fighting a spiritual battle. The enemy tells us we will fail, but we can't listen to him or succumb to fear. Instead, we must listen to the voice that tells us that we *can* do it. God heard my wife and I when we cried out to Him in our living room, and He will hear your cry as well.

Steve Reynolds

Man Up

Eat Up: 35 a Day

Fiber fights off fat, so if you want to live a long, productive, high-energy life, eat high-fiber foods such as beans, lentils, vegetables, fruits, nuts and whole grains. Research has shown that people who eat fiber not only lose fat but also lower their cholesterol and avoid diabetes, heart disease and even some cancers. In addition to these benefits, fiber fills you up so you don't eat as much, gives you long-lasting energy, boosts your immune system and improves bowel regularity. Work up to eating 35 grams of fiber each day.

Pump Up: Gladiator Gluts

Begin by lying on your back. With your knees bent, bring your feet together flat on the ground at a 90-degree angle to the ground. Sit with your palms flat on the ground with your fingertips pointing toward your heels. Lift your hips off the ground while pressing your arms into the floor. Squeeze your gluts together, lift your hips, and release by bringing your hips down to the floor. Do a set of 10, rest, and repeat. Go for as many reps as possible.

Reflection and Discussion Questions

1. Tom Landry once said, "Setting a goal is not the main thing. It is deciding how you will go about achieving it and staying with that plan." What does this mean to you in terms of getting on track to a healthier lifestyle?

2. How many of Satan's Seven Deadly Lies have you heard him whisper in your ear? Number the following in the order in which they are the most problem to you, with #1 being the most difficult to deal with and #7 the least difficult.

___ Lie #1—Failure: You're not going to succeed.
___ Lie #2—Time: You don't have time to lead a healthy life.
___ Lie #3—Fear: You might hurt yourself (or even die!).
___ Lie #4—Denial: You don't *really* have a problem.
___ Lie #5—Blame: It's not your fault.
___ Lie #6—Difficulty: It's too hard for you.
___ Lie #7—Emotions: You won't feel better about yourself.

3. Look at the lie you identified as being the most difficult to overcome. What truths from the Bible given in this lesson helped you?

4. Now that you have identified the toughest lie to overcome, write out a prayer asking God to help you overcome it.

    _____
    _____
    _____
    _____
    _____

5. What are five things you can do when Satan comes to you with this lie (such as pray, read the Bible, and recite God's promises)? Remember that you are an overcomer through Jesus Christ.

    1. _____
    2. _____
    3. _____
    4. _____
    5. _____

6. In Romans 8:5, Paul says that if you are going to live according to the Spirit, you must first think according to the Spirit. Reading your Bible will help you think this way. What can you do to spend more time in God's Word?

    _____
    _____
    _____
    _____
    _____

MY PERSONAL GAME PLAN FOR

GETTING IN SHAPE

*Beloved, I pray that you may prosper in all things
and be in health, just as your soul prospers.*
3 JOHN 2

This book is about **ACTION** and about **DOING**! In the spaces below, record what actions you are going to take to improve your health this week.

Aware—I will do the following to show I am aware of my current physical condition and that my body matters to God:

_____

_____

_____

_____

_____

Commit—I will do the following to commit to living a disciplined life and to winning over temptation:

_____

_____

_____

_____

_____

_____

Transform—This is how I will transform the way I think and live:

_____

_____

_____

_____

_____

Incorporate—I will incorporate these healthy eating habits and exercise into my daily life:

_____

_____

_____

_____

_____

Organize—This is how I will organize a team of people to help me win:

_____

_____

_____

_____

_____

Navigate—This is my action plan for healthy living and navigating my way to leaving a lasting legacy:

_____

_____

_____

_____

_____

Chapter 6

Progress, Not Perfection

*Therefore we also, since we are surrounded by so great a cloud of witnesses,
let us lay aside every weight, and the sin which so easily ensnares us,
and let us run with endurance the race that is set before us.*

HEBREWS 12:1

Picture this: a guy is sitting on the couch on Sunday afternoon wearing his favorite team jersey. He's screaming at the TV and the players on the field. He yells to his wife, "Hey, honey! Bring me the chips and a drink . . . and don't forget the dip!"

"Get it yourself!" she yells back.

"I can't get up!" he answers over the roar of the TV. "I might miss a big play!"

How many times have you been watching a football game and found yourself on the edge of the couch waiting for that one big play? The Hail Mary pass to the endzone to win it all. The long-distance field goal just as time runs out. The 99-yard pass play or kickoff return that goes all the way. The interception and runback to score the winning touchdown. Those plays are amazing! They get the adrenaline pumping.

But honestly, guys, how often do those plays happen? How many games are really won by the "big play"? In fact, as of the writing of this book, there have only been *13* successful 99-yard pass plays in NFL history.[1] By far, more games are won by one team methodically pushing the ball yard-by-yard down the field at a slow and steady pace. They are won with players who have their heads in the game who are focused on reaching their goals through incremental steps. This is where your focus needs to be right now as well. You need to stop waiting for that "big play" in your life. There isn't a magic pill that is going to completely erase all of your health issues, concerns and all those extra pounds. There isn't a magical contraption that for four easy payments of $19.99 is going to vibrate the fat right off your belly. (Don't laugh, guys—years ago I actually bought a device like this.) There are no Hail Mary passes when it comes to your health.

Remember, you didn't get this way overnight, and you aren't going to erase the damage from years of neglect overnight either. It's going to take time, hard work and developing new habits and routines that produce lasting change. Men, your new battle cry has to become *"Progress, NOT perfection!"* It's all about getting rid of the bad habits that are weighing you down, just as the author of Hebrews 12:1 states.

Think of yourself as the quarterback of a football team. Your job is to slowly move the ball down the field to your endzone. You do that by grinding it out, one play at time, to slowly start producing change in your life. In the beginning it may feel as if you aren't making any progress, but don't give up—you are now in the game now and you will start seeing results. Remember, your goal is to just start seeing progress, so don't focus on perfecting everything right away. If you keep working at it and drilling down on each new play that you implement in your life, you will eventually reach your goals and have success.

Stop Procrastinating

But first, you have to stop procrastinating and putting off taking care of your health. The bottom line, guys, is you have to start *sometime* . . . so why not start *today*? James teaches this very idea in your ultimate Playbook, the Bible:

> Whereas you do not know what will happen tomorrow. For what is your life? It is even a vapor that appears for a little time and then vanishes away. Instead you ought to say, "If the Lord wills, we shall live and do this or that." But now you boast in your arrogance. All such boasting is evil. Therefore, to him who knows to do good and does not do it, to him it is sin (James 4:14-17).

In these verses, James tells you that there is no promise that you will see tomorrow. Your life is like a vapor; you could be here today and gone tomorrow. For this reason, you can't put off things you should be doing today. Not only do you have to stop procrastinating, but you also have to start doing those things that you know are right. If you don't, you are sinning against God and your body, the temple of the Holy Spirit.

So reject procrastination. Say to yourself, *I am no longer going to put off what I could start today. I am going to begin my new life. I am going to make the changes I need to make. I am going to quit making excuses for my failures and for the sorry choices I am making in my life. I am not going to grow weary in doing well. I am going to move forward in my life and change my future by changing what I do today.*

Stop Making Excuses

For true change to occur in your life, you have to stop making excuses. This is a tough one! After all, you've likely worked hard to come up with some good excuses for why you can't get up and exercise and start eating healthier. Over the years, I think I've heard them all. Here are just a few of the ones I hear often:

- I'm too tired.
- My bones hurt.
- I deserve a break after everything I have been through today.
- Why get up? It won't matter.
- It's too cold.
- It's too hot.
- It's too late in the day.
- It's too early in the day.
- It might rain. I'm sure the weather will be better tomorrow.
- I just ate.
- It's too far to drive to the gym.
- I don't want to miss a minute of my favorite TV show.
- Everyone is going to be talking about the game tomorrow, and I don't want to look like an idiot because I didn't watch it.
- I have my good clothes on, and I am not going to change.
- What good is a man-cave if you can't get any use out of it?
- I shouldn't have to exercise. After all, my friend's wife lets him stay on the couch during football season!
- I'm already married. Who do I have to look good for and impress?
- My job takes too much of my time. I don't have time to work all day, spend time with the wife and kids, and also have time for a workout.
- I'm too old to change. Can't teach an old dog new tricks.
- I'm too fat to exercise.
- I hate to sweat.
- I just don't feel like it.

Excuses, excuses, excuses. I'm sick of them. Are you? They are like those annoying commercials that interrupt the flow of the game. I mean, really, who wants to watch a commercial about car insurance right when your team has gotten possession of the ball? I certainly don't. Excuses are interruptions, and if you don't get rid of them, they will interrupt the flow of your life. No more commercial interruptions.

The reality is that excuses are built around bad habits. The *real* reason you don't want to exercise is because you want to sit around and watch TV. You don't want to wake up a little earlier to exercise and pack a healthy lunch because you stayed up too late the night before. You don't *want* to change your old routines in order to incorporate more healthy ones. But if you are going to overcome the huge obstacle of procrastination, you have to overcome those bad habits that have become so engrained in your brain. They are like those old clothes you've had in the closet for years that you just can't bear to part with.

I have an old T-shirt and shorts that I love to wear when I am relaxing at home. My family thinks they are pretty gross, and if I were honest with myself, I would have to agree with them. They are old and faded and have stains on them from food I've spilled on myself while eating. They don't smell very good, because they rarely ever make it into the laundry. They certainly aren't attractive, and they don't make me look good. I wouldn't wear them out to dinner or to work. But they sure are comfortable, and I love to put them on after a hard day's work. It's not like they are my only options to wear at home; I just like wearing them. It would be hard to part with them.

Your bad habits are just like my old stinky, smelly, ugly T-shirts. They don't make you look good, and I bet they don't make you feel good about yourself. In fact, you would probably be embarrassed if you had unex-

Check Up

Big Belly = Low Testosterone
In men, being overweight or obese is strongly linked to lower levels of testosterone. This can have many serious health ramifications, as low testosterone levels are known to be associated with erectile dysfunction, hypertension and depression. It is believed that excess fat cells metabolize (convert) testosterone to estrogen, causing both lower testosterone levels and higher estrogen levels in men, which, in turn, causes mood lability (unstable and likely to lapse or change), gynecomastia (breast development), and lower sex drive and performance.

pected guests stop by who caught you doing those bad habits. It's time to throw them out. It's time to start acting like the valuable player you truly are. It's time to throw out the old and adopt the new. It's time to produce change in your life so that you can finally be rid of those old habits.

Producing Change

As I've stated, you have to start thinking of yourself as a work in progress. This means that your work will never truly be complete. This is the first thing you have to wrap your head around when trying to figure out how to produce change in your life: you are to be engaged in a process of *constant change*. I love how Paul describes this in Colossians 3:8-10:

> But now you yourselves are to put off all these: anger, wrath, malice, blasphemy, filthy language out of your mouth. Do not lie to one another, since you have put off the old man with his deeds, and have put on the new man who is renewed in knowledge according to the image of Him who created him.

This is an incredible passage of Scripture in which Paul describes how you must put off the old and put on the new. If you want to maximize your health and your life, you need to be in a constant state of change by putting off your old bad habits and putting on new good ones. Think of those old habits as weights that are slowing you down and keeping you from running toward the goal. Listen once again to what the author of the key verse in this chapter has to say about laying all those weights aside:

> Therefore we also, since we are surrounded by so great a cloud of witnesses, let us lay aside every weight, and the sin which so easily ensnares us, and let us run with endurance the race that is set before us (Hebrews 12:1).

You can't be weighed down by sin and those stinky old habits. Instead, you have to run with endurance so that you can finish strong. But how do you do this? How do you let go of those things that are slowing you down and defeating you? Let's take a look at four points about change you need to know in order to do this.

Point #1: Change Is Supernatural

In 2 Corinthians 5:17, Paul says this: "Therefore, if anyone is in Christ, he is a new creation; old things have passed away; behold, all things have become new." The change Paul is referring to here is a supernatural change. It is a change that God makes in your life and in your heart.

This change occurs when you grow and develop your relationship with God and start going deeper with Him. When you are in Christ—when your life is centered on Him—a supernatural change begins to take place in you from the inside, not the outside. God begins to move, and suddenly you are on the way to becoming a new creation. But before this can happen, you have to admit that you can't change without God. You have to come to the end of yourself and realize that if change is going to happen, you need His help. You have to say to yourself, *It is not about self-control. It is not about doing better. It is not about trying harder. It's not about anything I can do, but what God can do in me.* You have to get to the place where you can say, *I give up. I can't do it. I can't change without God. I have got to get in Christ.* Then you have to believe that you *can* change through God.

In Jeremiah 32:27, God says, "Behold, I am the LORD, the God of all flesh. Is there anything too hard for Me?" There is nothing too hard for God! He can help you change. You just have to say to yourself, *Let go, and let God!* Say that out loud right now: "Let go, and let God." Then really let go of the old things—your old habits—and allow God to change you from the inside out.

So, the next time you are tempted to put on that stinky old habit of pulling into a fast-food restaurant and ordering your favorite value meal, pray that God will give you the strength to put on a new habit. Ask Him to help you put down the remote when you come home from work and go for a bike ride instead. Pray that He will give you the strength to wake up earlier in the morning so you can pack a nutritious lunch and snacks for the day. Or pray that He will help you make better food choices if you have to eat out. These are new habits that you need to develop, and you need God's help to do them.

Point #2: Change Is Mental

In the last chapter, we discussed how you need to get your head in the game and change the way you think, but the point is worth repeating here. Change *begins in the mind*. It starts with the way you think. So, in order to produce change, you have to do some things that will exercise your mind.

Read the Bible Every Day

The first thing you have to do is put the lies Satan tries to use against you out of your mind by reading your Bible every day and meditating on the truth you find within its pages. You have to read the Bible, memorize it, listen to it and live it every day. Only then can you change the way you think and act. In Ephesians 4:22-24, Paul says:

> Put off, concerning your former conduct, the old man which grows corrupt according to the deceitful lusts, and be renewed in the spirit of your mind, and . . . put on the new man which was created according to God, in true righteousness and holiness.

You must put off the old conduct that is corrupting you—the old way you lived and acted—and renew your mind by meditating on those things that are righteous and holy. So start reading something from the Bible every day.

Reject Negativity
The next thing you have to do is stay away from negative people—those individuals who bring you down and make you believe you can't win. Later on in the book we will discuss how you can build a team of people around you who are going to help you succeed, but for right now just focus on keeping these types of negative people at arm's length. Think of them as players on the opposing team. They are trying to distract you and to keep your eyes off the goal. Don't let them.

Get into a Good Church
You also need to get into a good church that teaches you the Word of God and how to apply it to your life. Going to church and worshiping with the Body of Christ will redirect your thinking and help you focus on God. It will help you take your mind off yourself and your problems and put it on God and His solutions. Man, when you are standing amongst a group of other believers singing and praising God, you begin to feel His presence, and it energizes you. Listening to sermons online or podcasts of messages is another great way of exercising your mind and training it to think on things that are holy and true. (You can visit our website at www.capital baptist.org and listen to our sermons. They are there to encourage you and to help you grow.)

Read Something on Health Each Day
Finally, make it a point to read something on health and wellness every day. Become an expert on living healthy. I try to spend at least 15 minutes each day doing this. It helps me stay focused on my goals, inspires me to try new things, and keeps me on track. I guarantee that you will find all

kinds of ways to incorporate new habits into your life if you spend just a little time every day educating yourself and growing in this area.

Point #3: Change Is Helpful

Change is flat-out helpful. Have you ever poured a bowl of cereal and, when you went to grab the milk carton from the fridge, found it empty? Or, worse, have you ever sat down on the toilet only to face an empty toilet paper roll? Certainly, change can enhance your quality of life!

Unfortunately, as men, we hate change. We drive the same way to work, we sit in the same seat at church, we like our coffee the same way we have always had it. We're not into all the lattes and frappes and mochachinos. We are creatures of habit, and you had better stand back if our sacred routines and rituals get interrupted. But we have to recognize that change *is* helpful. In Galatians 6:7-9, Paul says this:

> Do not be deceived, God is not mocked; for whatever a man sows, that he will also reap. For he who sows to his flesh will of the flesh reap corruption, but he who sows to the Spirit will of the Spirit reap everlasting life. And let us not grow weary while doing good, for in due season we shall reap if we do not lose heart.

This important passage of Scripture contains what I believe to be the most important and powerful law in all the world. It is a law that none of us can escape and one that every one of us must embrace, because whether we acknowledge it or not, we are going to live it. It is called the law of *sowing and reaping*.

This is an agricultural term used in farming, and it means that whatever you sow, you will reap. For instance, if you want to have corn, you have got to sow corn. If you want to have strawberries, you have to sow strawberries. If you want to live a healthy life, you have to sow healthy habits. The Bible is clear that if you sow to your flesh, you will reap corruption. That is what I did in my life—I ate what I wanted to eat, never exercised, and sowed to my flesh. And what did it do? It corrupted my body. But when I began to sow to the Spirit, I started to reap new life.

It's simple: *The decisions you make will determine your destiny.* For the most part, you are where you are today because of the decisions you have made or the decisions that others have made for you. You are where you are because of the choices you made in the past. So, here is the deal: If you want to change your life and change what you are reaping, begin to sow the correct things into your life. Don't forget the promise found in Galatians 6:9:

"Let us not grow weary while doing good, for in due season we shall reap if we do not lose heart."

Change is helpful because (1) it will decrease your pain, and (2) it will increase your pleasure. If you are making positive changes in your life in regard to your health, change will reduce the pain that comes with being obese and overweight while producing pleasure in feeling better, looking better and having a better outlook on life. In Psalm 16:11, David says to God, "You will show me the path of life; in Your presence is fullness of joy; at Your right hand are pleasures forevermore." Isn't that good? In God's presence is the *path of life*. In God's presence is *fullness of joy*. In God's presence are *pleasures forevermore*. So start sowing good, healthy habits into your life and routines, and you will reap a healthier and more productive life.

Point #4: Change Is Possible

Finally, you have to understand that change is possible. In Romans 8:31, Paul says, "What then shall we say to these things? If God is for us, who can be against us?" Doesn't that get you pumped up? It pumps me up.

Always remember that God is your Coach and that He is for you. He wants you to win. Do you understand that? *He is for you.* He doesn't want you to waste your life; He wants you to maximize it. He wants to help you produce change. He wants to give you the strength you need to change those bad habits that are slowly killing you. He wants to inspire and encourage you with His Word. He wants to speak truth into your life. Nothing is too hard for Him. You just have to trust that with God, change *is* possible.

In action movies, we all love it when the good guys win. The cool thing is that God is a conqueror, and through His help, you can be a conqueror as well. You can fight the battle of overcoming all those bad habits and excuses so you can be victorious. All things are possible with God. So stop making excuses and start taking action today.

Start Small to Win Big

I love the fable of *The Tortoise and the Hare*. Even though it's a children's story, the lesson it teaches is such a vital one for us at this stage of the game. Even though the hare was much faster than the tortoise, he kept getting distracted along the race and kept losing sight of the finish line. The tortoise, on the other hand, never lost sight of the goal. He kept moving at a slow and steady pace until he reached the finish line ahead of the hare.

I love the moral of the fable: *Slow and steady wins the race.* Keep that in mind, guys, as you are transforming your routines and habits. Start slow, start small, and don't lose sight of the finish line. Pick one positive thing you can do today to get started. Maybe you can drink more water today or go for a walk. Maybe you can park a little farther away from your office or store, or, better yet, determine to limit the number of times you go through the drive-thru. Get out of the car and walk in. I'm sure if you were honest with yourself, there are many small steps to life you could take that would help kick-start the momentum you need to start producing positive change. (In my first book, *Bod4God: The Four Keys to Weight Loss,* you can read more about the small steps to life that I took to help me improve my health and quality of life.)

Picture a baby learning to walk. He or she starts with slow, small steps that at first are a little wobbly, unstable and uncertain. Well, it's time to start learning to walk a new walk right now. It's time to start with those small baby steps and use them to lead you to new, healthier habits.

Now that you have begun your *transformation*, in the next two chapters, we will be looking at ways you can start to *incorporate* simple changes into the way you look at eating and exercise. Think of these tips as new plays that you will be practicing and trying out. Some may work for you, and some may not. That's okay; after all, not every new play a football coach goes over with his or her team works perfectly the first time. Plays have to be tweaked and refined, which is what you need to do next: find out what works for you and your new lifestyle. Also, don't forget that we are working for progress, *not* perfection.

So keep moving that ball down the field until you reach your endzone. Grind it out, and push hard. If you do, you will soon find that you are off and running down the field on the heels of lots of new habits that you have sown into your life. In the next two chapters, we'll discuss how to *incorporate* those changes to create a better life.

Chris Wilcox
The Fat Joke Was on Me

LOST 223 POUNDS

Before	After

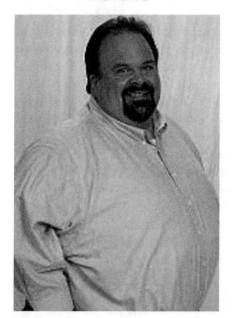 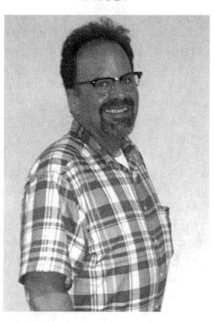

When my weight reached 451 pounds, I couldn't see over my belly, so I bought a talking scale. I was a one-man lawn-furniture destruction crew. I do stand-up comedy, but at 451 pounds, most of my jokes were fat jokes. I like to make people laugh, but the truth is that I felt hopeless and guilty for my condition.

I ate anything and everything. In restaurants, I always ordered the largest thing on the menu. It was never about taste, but simply about quantity. I ate from the time I got home from work until I went to bed at three or four in the morning. I was missing out on life and on spending time with my family and friends, because I had simply gotten too big to be comfortable anywhere but in my favorite chair. I couldn't go up the stairs without getting completely out of breath. I had tried everything to lose weight, including surgery, but I was just as big as ever. My weight just kept creeping up.

What finally caught my attention happened sort of on accident. *The Biggest Loser* reality show came to Washington, DC, and the producers were interviewing candidates for their next season. I tried out for the show not because I had confronted the reality of my weight problem but because I thought it would be good for my stand-up career. As it turns out, I didn't make it onto the show, but I did progress far enough to be called for an on-camera interview.

That interview proved to be a turning point and showed how real the participants' emotions on that show really are. The producers asked me questions that I had never thought to ask myself. They asked if my comedy would seem funny if told by a fit person, or if it would just seem mean. They asked if I thought people were really laughing *with* me or just *at* me. They asked what my children might be thinking when they saw me eating myself to death. I wept.

When I got home from the audition, I went for a walk. I walked about a block before my huffing and puffing forced me to stop. I turned around to go home and found that the way home was uphill. I couldn't do it.

Later on, I went to my friends on Facebook and posted my story. Those folks became my greatest encouragers, and they still are to this day. I began to take small steps to life as suggested by Pastor Steve in *Bod4God: The Four Keys to Weight Loss*—not huge things, but just simple things I could do to get more exercise.

The small changes I made worked pretty quickly. I began losing two to three pounds each week, and those successes encouraged me to keep going. To date, I've lost 223 pounds, and I'm two-thirds of the way to my goal weight of 180 pounds.

Another small step I took was to get rid of all pre-packaged food in my house. I changed from eating red meat to eating mostly chicken and fish. I haven't had a cheeseburger in two years, but I do eat turkey burgers. Another simple change I made was to eat five times a day. Yes, you read that correctly: *five times*. Here are some sample meals I eat each day:

- **Breakfast:** Two slices of whole-grain toast with-lean turkey and an egg on top, and a slice of 2% cheese.

- **Mid-morning snack:** a 100-calorie snack of almonds.

- **Lunch:** An apple, a stalk of celery and carrot snack-pack, and a package of crackers with cheese. I also often indulge in a weakness—two 40-calorie Slim Jim sausage sticks. (By this time, I have accumulated about 900 calories for the day.)

- **Afternoon snack:** a 90-calorie Kashi® bar.

- **Dinner:** lean ground turkey, fish, or chicken and vegetables. (By the end of the day, I have taken in about 1,800 to 2,000 calories. Based on that amount of calories, I can lose two to three pounds a week.)

I go to the gym three days each week, where I do cardio exercise and low-rep weight training, lifting to point of failure. Although you don't have to go to a gym, I like to do so because I can work out with my accountability buddy—my son. (I like to refer to him as my "acountabili-buddy.") Note that I didn't start out by making losing 223 pounds my goal; rather, I set interim goals and reset them about every six weeks—15 pounds by the next goal setting date. If I didn't make my goal, I knew I had done something wrong, and I usually knew what that was.

I have a new role in life, and it is as an encourager. So let me encourage you. Losing weight has huge positive benefits. It's a way to get your life back. You'll feel better and look better. Your clothes will fit differently, and after a while they won't fit at all. That means you'll have to get some new duds! I recently pulled out a pair of shoes I hadn't worn in a long time, and guess what? They were too big. I didn't know it, but you not only lose weight around your middle but also in your feet and hands. Hey, that too-tight wedding band is trying to tell you something, and you'd better pay attention.

Man Up

Eat Up: Read the Fine Print

Reading food labels will lead to losing weight. You can still enjoy some of your favorites while you lose weight if you start comparing labels and pick those products with the fewest calories, sugar, salt, fat and artificial ingredients per serving. Again, most of what you want to be eating for long-term health won't even have a label. Focus on filling up first with fruits, vegetables, whole grains, beans, nuts, fish and lean meats.

Pump Up: Shoulder Shredders

Doing shoulder circles is great for working the entire shoulder girdle, even the tiny muscle fibers. This exercise ensures a full-blown shoulder workout. Stand with your feet shoulder-width apart, with arms extended from both sides and your palms down. Keeping the arms extended, begin moving them in a forward circular motion. Keep the movements small and tight. Progress to a larger and looser circular range of motion. Do as many circles as you can, and then rest and change rotation direction.

Reflection and Discussion Questions

1. What comes to mind when you hear the phrase "progress, not perfection"?

   _____

   _____

   _____

   _____

2. What would your life look like if you refused to procrastinate about your health?

   _____

   _____

   _____

   _____

3. Review the list of excuses people make for not changing their unhealthy lifestyle habits. Which one sticks out in your mind? How have you used this to rationalize that you do not need to lead a healthier life?

   _____

   _____

   _____

   _____

4. In what ways have you resisted change in your life? What changes do you need to make to start leading a healthier life?

   _____

   _____

   _____

   _____

5. In this chapter, we discussed how change is supernatural, how it begins in the mind, how it is helpful, and how it is possible. Which of these points stands out the most to you, and why?

_____

_____

_____

_____

_____

6. The author of Hebrews 12:1 tells us to lay aside everything that is hindering us from running "the race that is set before us." What specific things do you need to put off in order to achieve your health goals?

_____

_____

_____

_____

_____

MY PERSONAL GAME PLAN FOR

GETTING IN SHAPE

*Beloved, I pray that you may prosper in all things
and be in health, just as your soul prospers.*

3 JOHN 2

This book is about **ACTION** and about **DOING**! In the spaces below, record what actions you are going to take to improve your health this week.

Aware—I will do the following to show I am aware of my current physical condition and that my body matters to God:

_____

_____

_____

_____

_____

Commit—I will do the following to commit to living a disciplined life and to winning over temptation:

_____

_____

_____

_____

_____

_____

Transform—This is how I will transform the way I think and live:

_____

_____

_____

_____

_____

Incorporate—I will incorporate these healthy eating habits and exercise into my daily life:

_____

_____

_____

_____

_____

Organize—This is how I will organize a team of people to help me win:

_____

_____

_____

_____

_____

Navigate—This is my action plan for healthy living and navigating my way to leaving a lasting legacy:

_____

_____

_____

_____

_____

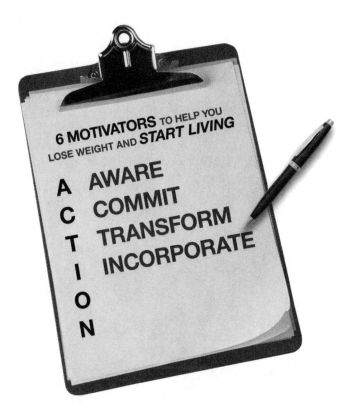

Incorporate

The fourth step in your journey toward getting off the couch and getting into shape is to **incorporate** healthy eating habits and exercise into your daily routines. It's time to put what we've been talking about into action and start making changes in how you eat and live your life. Start thinking of food as fuel, and start feeding your body healthy living food. You won't reach your goals sitting on the couch eating junk—you have to *get up* and *get moving*. If you do, you will begin to see results, and your body will thank you.

Chapter 7

Get Buff, *Not* Buffeted

And put a knife to your throat if you are a man given to appetite.
PROVERBS 23:2

"Pastor Steve, I'm sitting at McDonalds with my Bible to my left and a copy of *Bod4God* in front of me," a pastor once wrote to me. "I just consumed two #2 combos and a sweet tea, and am now I'm enjoying a coffee. I am another overweight shepherd in God's Church. Steve, I write to you out of desperation. At the age of 26, I currently weigh in at 324 pounds, just six years after weighing in at 215."

Fast food—or *fast death*, as I like to call it—plays a huge role in the obesity problem we are facing today in our culture. Americans (men in particular) are caught up in a fast-food frenzy. In this chapter, we will look at the consequences of this problem in our nation and what we can do to avoid it.

Men and Fast Food

It is a well-known fact that men are more likely than women to eat fast food, and it was certainly a way of life for me. As a pastor, I took advantage of every minute of my work day. I worked long hours and packed my time with appointments, meetings, visits and studying. Eating healthy was the *last* thing on my mind. I had too much to do, and people were counting on me. I had places to go and people to see. It was so easy to just hit the closest drive thru, order a quick lunch (something huge, because who knew how long it would be before I could take another break to eat), and devour my purchase while driving to my next destination. Most likely, I was on the phone the whole time I was doing this. The things I had to do were more important to me than the quality of what I was eating. And I'm not alone. In fact, recently I was shocked to learn that Americans spend nearly $100 billion on fast food *every year*.[1]

Finally, after examining what I was putting in my body every time I ate this stuff, I realized I had to adopt a new attitude. I have a friend who has a saying: "Avoid the colonel, the clown, the king and the queen, and even the red-headed girl who doesn't look mean." This had to become my new slogan. And while I applaud the effort that many fast-food places are now putting into offering healthier options, because the temptation to eat the unhealthier choices is so strong, I still advise people to drive *by* these restaurants, not *thru* them.

Not only did I like my food fast, but I also liked a lot of it. Just think of buffets. I used to love them. I was a big man with a big appetite, and buffets were as fast as a fast-food joint. When I walked into the restaurant, the food was ready, piping hot and just waiting to be consumed—and all at one great price! It was the greatest bang I could get for my buck. But I had to adjust my thinking about these places as well and realize that "buffet" really stood for **B**ig **U**nhealthy **F**at **F**olks **E**ating **T**ogether. As Proverbs 23:2 states, I was a man given to appetite, and there was no beating around the bush that buffets were leading me to eat too much unhealthy food.

If I wanted to lead a healthier life, I needed to adopt the mindset of athletic programs across the country that take a serious approach as to what their athletes eat. At the University of Nebraska, for example, trainers realized that proper fueling before and during competition could maximize their athletes' physical development and give them the competitive advantage they needed to succeed. They considered nutrition to be such a vital component of optimum sports performance that they actually provided a "training table" for their athletes. As an article on the university's website explains:

> The training table first opened in 1985 and currently offers lunch and dinner meals for student-athletes. The training table prides itself in providing the highest quality foods for athletes to enhance performance. All the foods served in the training table are labeled with a specialized food labeling system that helps athletes understand what foods they need to consume and the appropriate quantities to meet their individual nutritional needs.[2]

The buffets I liked to frequent at my favorite restaurants might have looked like a training table, but they were anything but. While I am sure there were healthy things on the menu, I didn't choose them. As I've mentioned before, most of us have a problem with portions, and I was no exception. With each pass at the buffet line there was always a hot, clean plate ready and waiting to replace the one I had just used, so there was nothing to stop me from gorging myself. It was just way too easy to eat too much of the wrong things. So I stopped going to them.

Have you ever ordered a dish at your favorite restaurant only to be astonished at its size when the waitperson delivered it to your table? I mean, holy cow, some dishes can feed four people, yet they are sold and served as a portion for one person. As Americans, we all suffer from portion distortion. We eat way too much food at one sitting. But we have to remember that the Bible says healthy living involves *eating less*. We have to make a conscious effort to eat smaller, healthier portions of food.

A Carton a Day

So, why do we still eat like this when we know it isn't good for us? The answer is because it is readily available, quick and easy. It's an addiction. Yes, you heard me—Christians may not be addicted to smoking pot, but we surely are addicted to potlucks!

Previously, I told you about my addiction: ice cream. While I didn't smoke a carton of cigarettes a day, I could certainly consume a carton of ice cream a day. When I look back on my old habits, I'm shocked by what I used to eat and how much of it I used to consume. Just as a drug addict demands more and more drugs to reach a place where he or she feels normal, my food addiction demanded that I eat huge amounts of food to come to a place of normality. That truly is an addiction.

I am from Virginia, and southern cooking was a way of life for me. I loved it! Sugar seemed to be the main ingredient in everything I ate. I grew up on fried chicken, biscuits, bologna gravy (that's right, *bologna* gravy), and pecan pie (*à la mode*, for sure). When Debbie and I married and started our family, these eating habits trickled down to my children. We also added some new things to our family menu—hot dogs, hot dogs and more hot dogs! They were cheap, quick and easy, and the kids loved them. Hamburger Helper was a household favorite and quickly became our best friend. After a long day of work, I could whip it up in a jiffy. We ate late because of my work schedule, and many times we ate from trays in front of the TV.

One of my favorite memories is of our frequent outings to 7-Eleven. I loved to take the kids there, and when we got inside, I told them they could each get one thing. There is very little at 7-Eleven that is healthy, and those outings were jammed-packed with calories, preservatives, sugar and all sorts of other things that were horrible for them. But it fed our craving for sweets and sugar. I was always right there in line with them, getting a Hershey bar or a Coca Cola Slurpee (one of my favorites). I loved sweets! I loved candy! In fact, truth be told, I even raided the children's church candy bin when I needed a quick fix for my sugar craving. How low is that?!

Jesus Is All for Food!

When I really started examining what I was eating, I went back to the Bible—my Playbook—for some guidance as to what I should or should not be eating. I mean, Jesus had to be pro food, right? He was human as well as divine, so He had to eat while He was here on earth. But *what* did He eat? I know He created the Milky Way, but I'm pretty sure He wasn't munching on Milky Way candy bars.

What I discovered is that even though the Bible does not tell us everything Jesus ate, food was on His mind and was a topic of concern during His ministry. He used food in His illustrations, as evidenced by parables such as the Sower and the Seed (see Matthew 13:3-9), Faith and the Mustard Seed (see Matthew 13:31-32), and the Great Banquet (see Matthew 22:2-14). He used wheat fields to depict a spiritual harvest that was ready to be reaped (see John 4:35). He performed miracles with food, such as the feeding of the 5,000 with five loaves of bread and two fish (see Mark 6:30-44). Another time, when the disciples were on the boat fishing, He told them to cast their nets into the water. They had caught nothing that day, but after following His command, they reaped an extraordinary take of fish (see Luke 5:1-7). Even Jesus' first miracle involved food, when He turned water into wine at a wedding feast in Cana (see John 2:1-11).

Check Up

Big Belly = Cancer Risk

The National Cancer Institute reports that obesity is associated with higher risks of certain cancer types, including cancers of the esophagus, pancreas, colon and rectum, kidney, thyroid and gallbladder. In 2007, approximately 34,000 cases of cancer in men were due to obesity. Researchers believe the reason for this high number is related to the fact that fat cells produce hormones called adipokines, which may adversely stimulate cell growth and lead to cancer. Studies have also shown a strong link between colorectal cancer and a sedentary lifestyle.[3]

Perhaps Jesus' most important illustration with food is the one He used with His disciples during their last Passover meal together to explain what would happen when He died on the cross. This is a practice that continues today in the taking of Communion, or the Lord's Supper (see Matthew 26:17-30; Mark 14:12-26; Luke 22:7-39; John 13:1-17:26). And just think about that great feast God has promised up in heaven at the time of the Marriage Supper of the Lamb (see Revelation 19:6-9). Jesus was all about food, and His desire is for us to be fit and healthy—not take our food away. He just wants us to make healthy choices when it comes to eating.

Not only did Jesus talk about food, but as a member of the Trinity, He also created food for us to enjoy. In Genesis 1:11, God the Father said, "Let the earth bring forth grass, the herb that yields seed, and the fruit tree that yields fruit according to its kind, whose seed is in itself, on the earth." In Genesis 1:29, He told Adam, "See, I have given you every herb that yields seed which is on the face of all the earth, and every tree whose fruit yields seeds; to you it shall be for food." These verses show that God wants us to enjoy the food we eat. He created us with an average of 10,000 taste buds and placed them along the path our food travels when we are eating it. Think about this for a moment. God chose to put those taste receptors—called *papillae*—in that location so we could enjoy the tastes of the wonderful foods He created for us to enjoy.

God's plan has always been for the bulk of our diet to come from "living food"—foods such as fruits and vegetables that are uncooked, unrefined and unprocessed. Hamburger Helper does not fit into this category, nor do chips, soda, cookies and candy. Many of these "dead foods" can last several years without going bad. If you don't believe me, just check out the "use by" date on a box of macaroni and cheese and see how long it can last. Manufacturers load up on preservatives and additives to keep it edible for an extended period of time.

It's time to clean house. Start by taking stock of the food you currently have. Survey how much of it is living food and how much of it is dead food. Get a garbage can, open the doors of your cupboards and pantry, and start tossing out the junk food. Get it out of your kitchen. *Start eating living food to live.*

A Recipe for Success

I've said it before, but it is so important that it bears repeating: We have to train ourselves to *eat for our health and not for our happiness.* I know this is tough to do, because so much of our culture revolves around food. Just think about the way marketers try to convince us that fast food will promote our happiness. IHOP has used the slogan, "Come hungry, leave happy." KFC has promised, "Buy a bucket of chicken and have a barrel of fun." Burger King has told us that "sometimes we've got to break the rules" and that we should be able to "have it our way."

We celebrate with food. We comfort with food. We bribe and reward with food. We even eat when we are bored and have nothing else to do. Disassociating food and feelings will be a total paradigm shift for most of us, but we have to let go of this "you deserve a break today" mentality that companies such as McDonald's want us to believe. Once again, if we are going to win the health game—and we must—we have to think of food as something that fuels our bodies, not our emotions. We have to start making changes in the way we eat and drink, and some of those changes, while not easy, will be necessary.

Water

I've said it before, but one of the easiest and least expensive changes you can instantly make is to start drinking more water. Just how much water do you drink? Are you even acquainted with H_2O? If you hang around me for any length of time, you will hear me say this repeatedly: "You must start drinking water immediately!" In fact, put the book down right now and go fill up a glass of clean, refreshing water. Take a drink. Isn't that great! Isn't that satisfying? Drink the rest of the water while you finish this chapter.

Water has been called the "solvent of life," as it is able to dissolve a wide range of substances. Some experts suggest that you need to ingest about half of your body weight in ounces of water every day to make up for what you lose through evaporation and waste.[4] (In other words, if you weigh 200 pounds, you need to drink 100 ounces of water per day.) Your body must have water to function, so it is important to continually replenish it. Just remember that if you were marooned on a desert island, you could live for about a month without food but only *three days* without water. Without water, your cells can't deliver oxygen to your tissues, your kidneys can't function properly, and your digestive can't break down food and absorb nutrients. *Water is crucial to healthy living!*

Dehydration, or the lack of water in our system, is a ferocious enemy to athletes, soldiers and all who work in the open air. Symptoms of moderate dehydration include dry mouth, little or no urine, sluggishness, a rapid heartbeat and lack of skin elasticity. Severe dehydration is a life-threatening condition characterized by extreme thirst, no urine, rapid breathing, altered mental state and cold, clammy skin. Dehydration can lead to a reduction in exercise performance and an inability to control body temperature, as well as difficulties in concentration, headaches, irritability, sleepiness and increases in body temperature and respiratory rates.[5] We live in a country with an abundant and pure water supply from the tap—a country where we don't have to go to the river with a five-gallon can on our head to get water that is marginally drinkable—so there is no reason we need to suffer these consequences. And yet we still choose to run around dehydrated because we don't consume the necessary amount of water that our bodies require.

For me, the biggest motivator in drinking more water was the fact that it aids in weight loss. In my mind, every time I drank a glass of water, I was washing the fat out of my body. It also helps tremendously in suppressing appetite. As Michele Stanton, fitness director for *Prevention* magazine, states, "If your body is even one-half cup shy of the amount it normally needs, your physical and mental energy will dip sharply."[6] So, the next time you start to feel a nagging desire to get a snack, drink some water instead. In fact . . . how are you doing with that glass of water? Drink it all!

Grilling

For some of you, drinking half your body weight in ounces of water each day will be a tough one to swallow. So let's talk about something positive. Guys, you don't have to give up the grill! You can cook healthy food that tastes great and at the same time do something you love. You just have to be careful what you are grilling.

Chicken, fish and lean beef are good choices for grilling. (Just make sure you cut off all visible fat.) Marinating your meat and adding spices and rubs to your favorite cuts can produce a tasty meal. You can grill vegetables to give them a delicious smoky taste. Try grilling red, yellow, orange or green peppers; onions; broccoli; asparagus; mushrooms; potatoes and all kinds of squash. Cut the vegetables thick so they don't fall through the grate, or skewer them kabob-style. You can also buy a grilling basket designed just for the purpose of grilling vegetables.

Grilling is a great way for you to share your newly adopted philosophy about food with your family and friends. Show them they don't have to give up taste for healthy eating. There are all kinds of resources and cooking aids out there on how to prepare really delicious meals using the grill. So strap on that apron, get the grilling tools out, and light up the coals!

Cold Cereal and Breakfast Bars

Most guys like to grab a bowl of cereal in the morning. The trick is finding a breakfast cereal that is healthy, low in sugar, has no trans fat and still tastes great. After all, if your cereal doesn't taste good you are probably not going to eat it, but some cereals are little more than sugar and refined white flour. Fortunately, there are some great healthy, good-tasting cereals out on the market, such as those made from toasted whole grains with nuts and dried fruit in them. Dried fruits add nutrition to your cereal.

When selecting a cereal, choose one that is high in fiber, as it will fill you up and keep you feeling full longer. Recent research among men aged 40 to 75 has found that adding bran to the diet reduced the risk of weight gain, while eating refined (or processed) grains had the opposite effect.[7] So again, look for cereals that are high in fiber and low in sugar.

Lots of guys like to grab a breakfast bar. But beware! Most bars are loaded with sugar and have little fiber. Read those labels (see the following section). It's okay to keep these bars around in case there's no time for breakfast, or as an emergency meal at the office or on a plane, but don't make eating them a habit. They are not nutritionally balanced enough to constitute a breakfast.

Whenever possible, choose a healthy bowl of hot oatmeal over a bowl of pre-packaged cold cereal. You can quickly microwave a bowl of oatmeal, and it will give you health benefits that will last a lifetime. Oatmeal is a cholesterol buster, is digested slowly by the body, and is high in complex carbohydrates. Sweeten your oatmeal with dried or fresh fruit, such as apples or raisins, and add milk. You can even add toppings such as flax, sunflower seeds, sesame seeds, almonds or walnuts to boost the nutritional value. Just avoid the pre-sweetened, chemical-coated single serving packs, as these miss the good stuff that sweeps your arteries clean.

My breakfast of choice is a small bowl of old-fashioned oats (not instant) with a handful of unsalted almonds and sweetened with Stevia. It fills me up and sticks with me through the morning. Other whole grains such as brown rice, whole wheat or corn-based hot breakfast cereals also deliver good health benefits. Brown rice-based cereals are cooked like oatmeal and are a great option for those who have wheat allergies. Brown rice has tons of fiber and is high in several minerals, including magnesium, phosphorous and potassium. Whole-grain brown-rice cereals can be found in your local health food store or in the health food section of your grocery.

Read the Label!

As previously mentioned, athletes at the University of Nebraska are taught how to read specialized labels so they can give their bodies the proper nutrition and the correct amount of food. In the same way, you have to begin learning how to read food labels. Americans are eating way too much processed food (more about that later) and have no idea what they are putting in their mouths—and they are reaping the consequences. If you want to break this pattern in your life, you need to know what you are eating. Your life depends on it.

In 1965, the Fair Packaging and Labeling Act was passed, which required all food manufacturers to "honestly and informatively" identify (1) the name of the product, (2) the place of business of the manufacturer, and, most importantly, (3) the type and amount of ingredients used in the product.[8] Since that time, further regulations by the Food and Drug Administration have refined what food manufacturers must include on their nutrition labels. For example, the following is a nutrition label for a Snickers Bar and an apple:

Nutrition Facts

Serving Size	1 Snickers bar 2 oz 57g (57 g)

Amount Per Serving	
Calories 271	Calories from Fat 122
	% Daily Value*
Total Fat 14g	21%
Saturated Fat 5g	26%
Trans Fat 0g	
Cholesterol 7mg	2%
Sodium 140mg	6%
Total Carbohydrate 35g	12%
Dietary Fiber 1g	5%
Sugars 29g	
Protein 4g	

Vitamin A	2%	•	Vitamin C	0%
Calcium	5%	•	Iron	2%

* Percent Daily Values are based on a 2,000 calorie diet. Your daily values may be higher or lower depending on your calorie needs.

Nutrition Facts

Serving Size	1 medium apple (154g / 5.5 oz.)

Amount Per Serving	
Calories 80	Calories from Fat 0
	% Daily Value*
Total Fat 0g	0%
Saturated Fat 0g	0%
Cholesterol 0mg	0%
Sodium 0mg	0%
Potassium 170mg	5%
Total Carbohydrate 22g	7%
Dietary Fiber 5g	20%
Sugars 16g	
Protein 0g	

Vitamin A	2%	•	Vitamin C	8%
Calcium	0%	•	Iron	2%

* Percent Daily Values are based on a 2,000 calorie diet. Your daily values may be higher or lower depending on your calorie needs.

Here's a quick lesson in how to read this label. As you read this information, remember that the big dangers to your health are fats, trans fats, sodium (salt) and sugar, so you especially need to know how much of those four substances you are putting into your mouth.

1. Begin by checking the *serving size* at the top of the label. Many individual packages have multiple servings. In this case, the Snickers bar is just one serving (one bar), as is the apple.

2. Check the total amount of *calories,* keeping in mind that an average man needs around 2,500 calories each day to maintain his weight. One Snickers bar has 271 calories, while one apple has 80. So, you could have three apples for the same calories in one Snickers bar. Which one would be more filling and keep you from getting hungry?

3. Check the *calories from fat,* which is listed to the right of the total calories. As you can see, a Snickers bar has 122 calories from fat, while the apple has none.

4. Check the total *fat* content. The Snickers bar has 14 grams of fat, while the apple has none. This column is further broken down by the amount of *saturated fat* (which raises bad cholesterol levels) and *trans fat* (which do double damage by raising bad cholesterol levels while lowering good cholesterol levels). The Snickers bar contains 5 grams of saturated fat and 0 grams of trans fat, while the apple has none.

5. Now look for the amount of *cholesterol* in the product. High levels of what is known as "bad" cholesterol can block arteries and lead to heart disease. The Snickers bar has 7 milligrams of cholesterol, while the apple has 1 milligram.

6. Check the *sodium* content. The lower the number, the better. A Snickers bar has 140 milligrams of sodium, while the apple has 1 milligram.

7. Check for total *carbohydrates,* which indicates the total of all the carbs in the product serving. The Snickers bar has 35 grams, while the apple has 22. High amounts of simple carbohydrates (such as those found in a Snickers bar) can lead to weight gain.

8. Check for *fiber*, which is important to maintaining good health. The Snickers bar has 1 gram of fiber, while the apple has 5 grams.

9. Check the *sugar* content in the product. The lower the number, the better. In this case the Snickers bar has 29 grams, while the apple has 16 grams.

10. Check the *protein* content. The amount of protein you need in your diet each day depends on your activity level. A 200-pound man who leads a sedentary lifestyle needs about 72 grams of protein per day, while a 200-pound athlete needs 126 grams per day.[9] The Snickers bar has 4 grams of protein, while the apple has none.

11. Finally, check the percent of daily nutritional values based on a 2,000-calorie per day consumption. The Snickers bar has 2 percent vitamin A, 0 percent vitamin C, 5 percent calcium, and 2 percent iron. The apple has 2 percent vitamin A, 8 percent vitamin C, 0 percent calcium, and 2 percent iron.

While nutrition labels for fruit vary according to size, all of the labels you find on apples will prove that it is a better choice for health than a Snickers bar.[10]

Processed Food

Let's look a bit more closely at some of this information on the nutrition label, focusing particularly on what we find in processed foods. "Processed foods" are those products you find in the center aisles of the store and much of what is in the freezer section. It is food that has been precooked and pre-prepared to make your life simpler. It is also a recipe for ruining your health. Here's why.

The majority of the American diet—perhaps as much as 80 percent—consists of processed foods that have been stripped of nutrients. While processed food is tasty, it is also loaded with additives and chemicals to make it look appealing and, more important to the manufacturer, give it a longer shelf life. These additives include sweeteners, salts, artificial flavors, factory-created fats, colorings, chemicals that alter texture and preservatives. If that isn't bad enough, the manufacturers strip out all the good stuff—soluble fiber, antioxidants, "good" fats—that protect your heart.

As I mentioned, the "biggies" to watch for in the nutrition labels are fats, trans fats, sodium (salt) and sugar, and you also need to pay attention to refined grains. Here is why these pose a greater problem to your health.

- *Fats:* How much fat you consume in your diet depends on your lifestyle, your weight, your age and your state of health, but the U.S. Department of Agriculture recommends most people keep their total fat intake at 20 percent to 35 percent of their daily intake of calories. Saturated fats, which are found in red meats and whole-milk dairy products, are especially problematic because they increase cholesterol levels, and should comprise no more than 10 percent of daily calories.[11] I recommend you limit eating red meat to once or twice per week. A cardiologist friend told me that smoking and hamburgers keep them in business.

- *Trans fats:* According to Harvard professor Walter Willett, introducing trans fats to our food is "the biggest food-processing disaster in U.S. history."[12] Trans fats are added to muffins, crackers, microwave popcorn and fast-food French fries. Even your supposed "heart-healthy" butter stick has trans fat. Trans fats clog arteries, causing an estimated 30,000 to 100,000 premature heart disease deaths each year. Furthermore, as previously mentioned, trans fats *boost* the levels of "bad" cholesterol while *decreasing* "good" HDL cholesterol. Replacing trans fats with good fats—such as fats found in olive oil, avocados, almonds, hazelnuts and peanut butter—could cut your heart attack risk by a whopping 53 percent.[13]

- *Sodium (salt):* Three-quarters of the sodium in our diets is found in processed foods such as canned vegetables and soups, condiments like soy sauce and Worcestershire sauce, fast-food and cured or preserved deli meats.[14] A recent shocker is the amount of salt in bread. Recent studies conducted by the Centers for Disease Control and Prevention reveal that a typical 1-ounce slice of bread has between 100 and 200 milligrams of salt, as compared to a typical 1-ounce serving of potato chips, which has 120 milligrams of salt.[15] Strive for less than 1,500 milligrams of salt per day.

- *Sugar:* High-fructose corn sugar is in almost everything we eat, including bread, bacon and even ketchup. Today, Americans consume nearly 63 pounds of it per person each year. Research is beginning to suggest that this liquid sweetener may raise the risk for heart disease and diabetes. It also encourages people to overeat, and it may also force the liver to pump more heart-threatening triglycerides into the bloodstream. To spot fructose on a food label, look for the words "corn sweetener," "corn syrup" or "corn syrup solids," as well as "high-fructose corn syrup."[16]

• *Refined grains*: Refined grains are all those white breads, pastas and sugary low-fiber cereals. These choices can boost your heart-attack risk by as much as 30 percent. Be careful even when choosing wheat flour or seven-grain varieties, as they may just be the same old refined breads the manufacturers have recast as "healthy." Check the label for amount of trans fat and note the first ingredient—on a healthy bread, it should be the grain used to make the bread. The fiber content should be at least 3 grams per serving.[17]

Some of these additives you will not find on the nutrition label for the food, but in the ingredients list—that little tiny print on the back of a package. So, if you truly want to know what you are putting in your mouth, you must read the ingredients list as well as the nutrition label.

Eating Out

One question that continually comes up whenever I discuss the topic of food is about eating out. I already told you how I feel about fast food, but to say that you will never eat out in any restaurant again is unrealistic. We are busy people, and eating out is more than likely going to be a part of our lives. As I've mentioned above, the trick is in making good choices about *where* you choose to eat out. For example, one restaurant serves a Bloomin' Onion, which is basically a large onion cut up to resemble a flower that is dipped in an egg wash, deep fried, and served with a large bowl of dipping sauce. Did you know there are 2,210 calories in that one appetizer alone?

This is not to say that there aren't a lot of good restaurants out there that have healthy choices on the menu. To help me make the best choices when eating in these establishments, I came up with an acronym: P-L-A-N. It's simple to remember, and it will really help you when you are looking at that menu. Here's the P-L-A-N:

Pray *consistently*. Pray that God will help you make wise choices and that He will strengthen you to keep that resolve to eat the healthy food your body needs.

Limit portions. Limit the size of what you are eating. If necessary, have your food server bring you a to-go box and pack up half the meal to take home before you start eating. It's a win-win situation: you limit what you are going to eat, and you have another meal ready for you to eat later at the same price.

Ask questions. I always ask lots of questions when at a restaurant. Is the fish grilled or fried? Do they put butter on the vegetables? Can they steam the vegetables for you? Do they have a smaller portion available? Educate yourself on the menu of your favorite restaurant and ask for healthy options.

No dessert. Finally, stay away from that dessert. You don't need it.

That's my P-L-A-N, and I'm sticking to it!

Embrace Technology

The last bit of advice that I want to leave with you is to embrace technology. With the availability of smartphones, iPads and other portable devices, many great resources that can help you succeed are now available right at your fingertips. Take some time to start researching them and looking for them. Now, I'm not going to give you a list of specific technologies to use—that is part of your homework for this chapter—but I will give you some ideas on things to look for that I believe will aid you.

First, with regard to your eating habits, look for apps or tools that help you track your food intake or calories consumed and burned in relation to your level of exercise. You can also find apps to help you plan healthy and nutritious meals, and apps to help you identify foods that are good or bad for you. One of my favorite resources is the First Place 4 Health website (www.fp4h.com), which provides taste-tempting, healthy, reduced-fat recipes for breakfast, lunch or dinner. Each recipe includes the nutritional information and serving size to help you make healthy choices when planning any meal. If you travel or eat out a lot, look for tools that list restaurants along with their menus so you can see the healthy options available to you at those places.

With regard to exercise, look for apps and other technologies that allow you to track the distance you run or walk, your heart rate, and the calories you are burning while exercising. You can also find tools to help you keep track of your exercise routine. Trust me, there are many helpful tools out there available for you to use. You just have to find the right ones for you.

It's Not a Diet, It's a Lifestyle Plan

Guys, even though we have talked a lot about food in this chapter, the main thing I want you to remember after reading this book is that this is *not about a diet, it's about creating a healthy lifestyle plan for you*. If I am repeating myself, I'm doing it for a reason. You have to find what works for you. Everybody is different, and what works for you might not work for another person. That's why I don't promote or push one single plan or approach to weight loss.

Take these thoughts, suggestions, tips and strategies that we have discussed in this chapter and start putting together a healthy eating plan that will work for you based on what the Bible says about food. Make a decision today that you are going to quit the fast-food frenzy and incorporate more living food into your diet. Get rid of soda and replace it with water. Take these simple steps, and you will see results.

Say, do you still have that glass handy? Before we deal with *incorporating* the dreaded E-word—*exercise*—into our plan, go fill up that glass again. Your body needs it.

Larry Kelley
Steps Back from the Banquet Table

LOST 62 POUNDS

Before	After
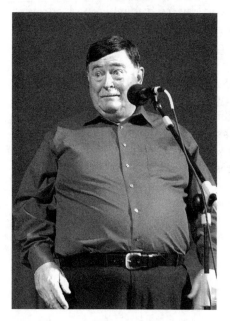	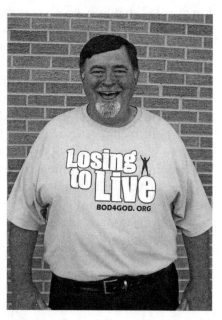

I have been overweight most of my life. I used to tell people that I was born at 10 AM, missed my first breakfast, and have been hungry ever since. Due to the extra pounds I put on, I began to hate words like "run," "rush" and "race," and I developed a strong love for words like "walk," "stroll" and "mosey." By the time I reached age 65, I was seriously overweight at 312 pounds.

You've probably heard it said that when you're trying to lose weight, you shouldn't skip breakfast—it is the most important meal of the day. Well, I wasn't skipping breakfast, I was skipping *to* breakfast. When I got up in the morning, the first thing that crossed my mind was, *I wonder what I can eat today*. The highlight of my day was consuming food. In 1 Thessalonians 4:4, Paul teaches that each of us should learn to control our own body in a way that is holy and honorable. We have the responsibility to control what we put into our bodies, but I wasn't doing that.

I am a professional storyteller from Chuckey, Tennessee. My wife, Gayleen, and I share stories at festivals, churches, schools, libraries, nursing homes and any other place where someone will listen. I have a Master's Degree in Storytelling from East Tennessee State University, and for 10 years I have taught there as a part-time adjunct storytelling instructor. My wife and I have always done a lot of travelling and public speaking—often for banquets. As a result, we consistently overate. When traveling, we would stop to eat at fast-food restaurants, and we just kept packing on the weight.

I thought that maybe I couldn't lose weight at my age, but then I read a story in my local newspaper about a faith-based weight-loss competition called "Losing to Live." It was being held at a Methodist Church in Johnson City, Tennessee, which was a round trip of 70 miles for us. When Gayleen and I entered the competition, the people there knew we were making a big effort to attend, and they treated us very well. We fell in love with them, the program and everything associated with it.

I had cracked a rib, and because of my weight it wouldn't heal properly. As a result of the rib and my big stomach, I couldn't get down to my feet to put my socks on. I felt pretty good about myself when I was storytelling, but the rest of the time I suffered from low self-esteem. That was the condition I was in when I entered the competition. I set a goal to lose 20 pounds during the 12 weeks of the competition. Surprise, surprise! By six weeks, I had lost 21 pounds. So I set a new goal. At 10 weeks, I had lost 30 pounds. By the end of the competition, I had lost 34 pounds, far exceeding any expectation I had ever had. Now I've settled down to a weight loss of about two pounds per week.

There are two small steps I now do that have continued to help me lose weight. One is portion size. I used to fill up a large bowl with cereal, but now I put my cereal in a cup. At the storyteller banquets I attend, I get a salad plate and use that for the food, rather than a large dinner plate. It's amazing how this helps control how much food I put into my body. The second thing I do is hike and walk. Since starting the Losing to Live competition, my wife and I have become walkers and hikers. On weekends we head out for a day hike on the Appalachian Trail, and during the week I regularly walk three miles a day. Recently, my wife and I hiked for five hours straight up the side of a mountain. Oh, what a view God had in store for us when we got there! This from a guy who couldn't get up the steps to the church.

It is wonderful that my wife is working with me on this. I tell folks, "We've been happily married for 32 years, mostly because she doesn't expect much out of me—and I have never disappointed her." Seriously, though, her biggest support has just been buying into the Losing to Live competition. Doing the competition together and supporting one another has been a wonderful gift. She is a cafeteria manager for little kids and she cooks all day, so I help cook at home. We eat lots of the veggies, fruits and other "living foods" that Steve advocates in the Losing to Live competition. Gayleen has diabetes, but after losing 20 pounds in the competition, her blood sugar has stabilized. I'm so proud of her.

Today, I like to encourage other seniors not to underestimate what God can do in their lives. With His help, we can lose unhealthy weight and have a better quality of life. There are many passages of Scripture relating to health that can encourage us. I also tell people not to underestimate the power of being part of a team, as it can give them support and accountability. Recently, my wife and I even decided to start a competition at Limestone Free Will Baptist Church, where we direct the seniors' ministry. Our first competition had 54 people in attendance. We are trying to involve not just seniors but also whole families, as weight problems usually run through an entire family.

I became a Christian at 34 years of age, and from that moment on I have never wanted to disappoint the Lord. Now that I've committed to lose the excess weight, I want to continue on so I can follow His instruction to care for my body. He's helping me. It's almost unbelievable, but He took away my love of a big bowl of ice cream and my desire for fast food. I've lost pounds before, but now I want to keep it going. It all boils down to my responsibility to continually ask God for help and to praise Him for the successes.

One thing that really touched me during the competition came from a testimony I heard on one of the *Bod4God* DVDs. A lady had lost a lot of weight, and when asked about how she had done it, she said, "First I had to lose the weight out of my heart." Think about it. Believing that we are too old, or that we not worth the effort, or any of the other lies of the devil are "weights in the heart." We have to lose these weights in order to succeed.

In closing, I want to offer you this promise: you will experience joy as you discover the fantastic life that God will give you when you can get up, go out, and see all that He has created.

Man Up

Eat Up: What Are You Drinking?

Today, think before you drink your calories. One of the easiest ways to lose weight is to limit your intake of calories from beverages. By switching to water, you might be able to lose five or more pounds in a week! So look at the calories in a serving of your favorite beverages such as soft drinks, energy drinks, sweetened fruit drinks, sports drinks, alcoholic drinks, teas and coffees. Just don't jump to artificially sweetened drinks, as research shows that these chemical additives are appetite stimulants and can cause you to actually consume more calories by the end of the day.

Pump Up: Strong-Man Squats

Squats are one of the best body-weight-bearing exercises a man can do. They work several areas, including the abs, legs, lower back and gluts. Begin by sitting in a chair and standing up. Do as many of these reps as you can—and then rest for 60 seconds. Add a backpack with books or a medicine ball for weight as you progress. To get an extra burn, try lowering your body and holding it a few inches above the seat of the chair for 5 to 10 seconds before returning to a standing position.

Reflection and Discussion Questions

1. What situation involving food is the most difficult for you to manage? Breakfast on the run? Eating out in a restaurant? Fast-food restaurants? Buffets?

   _____

   _____

   _____

   _____

2. It is important to drink about half of your body weight in ounces of water each day. Are you drinking enough water? If not, what steps will you take to drink more?

   _____

   _____

   _____

   _____

3. Are you taking the time to read nutrition labels before putting things in your mouth? If not, what will you do to make sure you do this important step?

   _____

   _____

   _____

   _____

   _____

4. In what ways are you using technology to manage your healthy eating?

   _____

   _____

   _____

   _____

5. After reading this chapter, how have you re-evaluated your eating choices and habits?

_____

_____

_____

_____

_____

6. Proverbs 23:2 says that overeating is serious business. What changes are you making to show you take this problem seriously?

_____

_____

_____

_____

_____

MY PERSONAL GAME PLAN FOR

GETTING IN SHAPE

*Beloved, I pray that you may prosper in all things
and be in health, just as your soul prospers.*
3 JOHN 2

This book is about **ACTION** and about **DOING**! In the spaces below, record what actions you are going to take to improve your health this week.

Aware—I will do the following to show I am aware of my current physical condition and that my body matters to God:

_____

_____

_____

_____

_____

Commit—I will do the following to commit to living a disciplined life and to winning over temptation:

_____

_____

_____

_____

_____

_____

Transform—This is how I will transform the way I think and live:

_____

_____

_____

_____

_____

Incorporate—I will incorporate these healthy eating habits and exercise into my daily life:

_____

_____

_____

_____

_____

Organize—This is how I will organize a team of people to help me win:

_____

_____

_____

_____

_____

Navigate—This is my action plan for healthy living and navigating my way to leaving a lasting legacy:

_____

_____

_____

_____

_____

Chapter 8

No Pain, No Gain!

But those who wait on the LORD shall renew their strength;
they shall mount up with wings like eagles, they shall run and not be weary,
they shall walk and not faint.

ISAIAH 40:31

"Exercise is the fountain of youth," says fitness expert Michele Stanton.[1] Nothing makes you look younger than a lean, healthy body. Hopefully, this will motivate you to start exercising again. At some point, you have to just do it! Exercise is probably going to be painful for you at first—both mentally and physically—but just remember: "No pain, no gain!"

I stared at those words on the wall of the weight room at Liberty University every day when I worked out. I didn't like them then, and I don't like them much better now, but they are true. You have to work *through* the pain to get *to* the gain. The good news is that the pain will lessen over time as your body adjusts to the new movement and exercise. You will grow stronger and stronger. That's the cool part. You can do it!

Surfing the Channels Is Not Exercise

Here's a newsflash: surfing the channels is not exercise. All those years I was sitting in my recliner relaxing, I didn't have one remote control for our TV, I had three—my three children. Getting up to change the channel would have at least been some sort of exercise, but that was too strenuous for me. I just had one of my kids change the channel, whichever one was closest to where I was sitting.

I should have been the one getting up to change the channels instead of telling my kids to do it. In fact, I shouldn't have been sitting there at all. I should have been up doing something, moving my body, taking better care of myself. But remember, I was the La-Z-Boy, not the chair, and I had made that deadly promise to myself to never exercise again. The idea that I had earned time to sit down and relax because I had worked hard all day was going to be a fierce opponent to overcome. I had become my own worst enemy.

Let's face it: most of us hate exercise, and while we are ready to *incorporate* changes into our diet, we are not ready to exercise. We would rather do anything than sweat. In America, we have adopted a decrease pain/increase pleasure mentality. Most of what we do centers around making ourselves comfortable. After all, none of us *likes* pain. We want comfortable cars, comfortable homes, comfortable furniture, comfortable clothes and comfortable shoes. We work toward building a retirement fund so we can live comfortably in our older years. We find pleasure in people, food, possessions, vacations, activities, spectator sports and all sorts of other things.

The only problem with this philosophy of life—this mentality—is that it is contrary to God's Word and His plan. In 2 Timothy 2:3, Paul tells us, "You therefore must endure hardship as a good soldier of Jesus Christ." Endure hardship? That doesn't sound like a whole lot of fun, but it is what we are commanded to do as followers of Jesus. We have to get this thinking out of our minds that everything is provided for our comfort. Yes, it will probably be painful to start exercising again, and it may not make us happy at first, but the end results will be worth it, and we will reap great gain in our lives.

Times Have Changed

The more I travel and talk to people across the country about the problem of obesity and being overweight, the more I am convinced that we have become a sitting culture. We simply don't need to move anymore, so we don't. We are flooded with resources and conveniences that have made our lives simple at the cost of keeping us active.

We can now cut the grass on our lawns on a riding lawn mower . . . or, better yet, can call one of those lawn-care companies to do it for us. We no longer need to change the oil in the car (in many urban areas, you're not even allowed to do it yourself). We can just drive into one of those 15-minute oil change places, and they'll do it quicker and more efficiently than we ever could. We do our banking at a drive-thru, get food and coffee at a drive-thru, get our car washed at a drive-thru, and fill our prescriptions at a drive-thru. In some places, we can even order our groceries online and have them carried inside our home. We've become a drive-thru, convenience-based society.

In this technological age, we spend much of our day on our backsides behind a computer or a desk. Many of us sit for hours in our cars while commuting to work. It's certainly common here in the D.C. Metropolitan area where I live. And if that wasn't enough, we sit when we get home. We spend hours and hours sitting in front of the TV or the computer. We play video games or watch movies instead of playing sports, riding bikes or doing other things outside. What happened to the days of bike races, street games, sandlot baseball, pickup basketball games and many other outdoor adventures?

So, what has all this sitting done to us as a society? Well, as Dr. James Levine of the Mayo Clinic has noted, "Researchers have linked sitting for prolonged periods with a number of health problems and premature death from cardiovascular disease."[2] For many of us, "sitting has become the new smoking."[3] Just let that sink in for a second . . . sitting is now being compared to smoking! Who would have thought that while we were making our lives easier and more convenient we were actually contributing to the downfall of our health?

When I stop and ponder these facts—when I look into the eyes of people who are in bondage to their current physical condition—I am deeply grieved. This is why I decided to do whatever I could to make a difference to bring about positive change to unhealthy and overweight people. This is why I have dedicated my life to helping them get moving and eating healthy. In my mind, it's a huge challenge, and one that can only be accomplished with Jesus' help. Jesus is our coach, and the Bible is our guide and Playbook.

You Say You Want to Be Like Christ?

I love the slogan, "**W**hat **W**ould **J**esus **D**o?" WWJD was an idea that started in the hearts of members of a small youth group. As people spoke those four simple words, it spread all over the world until it became a cultural phenomenon. It became a compass for their lives. But just what *did* Jesus do when it came to being physically active?

We don't know a lot about Jesus' early years at home with Mary and Joseph. We do know that His earthly father, Joseph, was likely a carpenter, and that Jesus took up the trade.[4] We never read that Jesus went looking for a way to exercise. However, as a carpenter, He more than likely had to lift heavy pieces of wood. He had to saw them into boards without power tools and pound pegs into holes He had drilled by hand without the use of a pneumatic nailer. Just imagine the strength He would have developed in his arms over the years. It was a movement-driven society.

Jesus was always on the move, particularly after He began His ministry. His whole life was exercise! The primary forms of transportation in His time were walking and taking a boat. Jesus and His disciples were not wealthy men who could own carriages, wagons or yachts. In fact, when Jesus sent them out in pairs, He told them to leave their worldly possessions behind and take only what they absolutely needed for the journey, because they were going to walk (see Luke 10:1-5). They walked through fields and valleys and up and down the mountains of that region.

Jesus, along with His disciples, must have been in great physical condition. They never had time to get out of shape. Just living their hard lives of manual labor and walking everywhere would have kept them conditioned. They did not have to consciously determine to exercise. But you do, and in the beginning it's going to be hard for you to get going. Think of it as if you were at training camp. Much of the ministry years of Jesus' life were a training camp for His disciples to get them ready for the future ministry they would have. Do you think it was easy for the disciples? Is it easy for all those pro football players? I think not!

Training Camp

When a player in the NFL attends a training camp, he joins with other players and coaches who have a common goal: winning the Super Bowl. The players are handed a schedule, and the first thing on the agenda is to

Check Up

Big Belly = Bad Joints
A study from the Johns Hopkins University Arthritis Center reports that a person who is 10 pounds overweight may increase the force on his or her knees and hips by 30 to 60 pounds with each step.[5] This leads to more injuries, more rapid joint deterioration and arthritis, which, in turn, leads to more joint pain, stiffness and swelling that often require complex orthopedic treatments (including medications, injections and surgeries). The outcomes of these orthopedic procedures are often not good, with higher risks of complications in obese individuals than in their non-obese counterparts. Chronic back pain is also associated with increased weight. Maintaining an ideal BMI and exercising regularly are the only proven modalities to slow the progression of joint arthritis.

meet with the head coach, staff, trainers and the team owner. The next morning, they practice from 9:00 AM to noon, have lunch, view a training film, and go back to the field for another two-hour practice. There are no outs, and no sidestepping the schedule. The players are required to be there, and they are required to work.

In a few days, the players get their pads, which weigh about 70 pounds. The team again goes through the whole practice routine, but this time each player carries those 70 pounds in 100-degree heat. This is where the players find out if they can survive the training. It is also where coaches see which players take being an athlete seriously and keep their bodies in top physical condition, and which players are lazy and don't work out. At this point, the athletes begin to understand that to play the game of football, they have to man up. They have to make the decision that if others can do it, they can do it too—and then they have to go for it.

More pain follows. After practice, the players shower and sit in tubs filled with ice water. It's a miserable experience, but the ice helps aching, swollen muscles recover like nothing else will. After dinner, another film and a snack, it is off to bed by 11:00 PM, because they have to be ready to do it all again tomorrow. The coaches take the curfew seriously, and they won't mess with players who don't get to bed on time. This is a player's life for the next six weeks. All this for a game.[6]

Training camp isn't easy for these players, and it is isn't comfortable for them. The same is true for us. In Matthew 16:24-25, Jesus said to His disciples, "If anyone desires to come after Me, let him deny himself, and take up his cross, and follow Me. For whoever desires to save his life will lose it, but whoever loses his life for My sake will find it." This passage of Scripture is repeated six times in the Bible, which indicates it is very important (see Matthew 10:39; 16:25-26; Mark 8:35-36; Luke 9:24-25; 17:33; John 12:24-26). It was a major theme of Jesus' teaching. He wanted people to know how to get life: by denying themselves, by taking up their cross, and by following Him.

Incorporating this Scripture into my life became the guideline for losing weight so I could live. In the same way, if you want to change your present physical condition and have health and a long life, you need to stand up, commit to doing something today, and find a training camp with other "players" where you can get the encouragement you need to take back control of your life. There is strength in associating yourself with a group of people who have goals that are similar to your own, and these individuals will help you succeed.

In 1 Corinthians 9:24,27, Paul writes, "Do you not know that those who run in a race all run, but one receives the prize? Run in such a way that you may obtain it. . . . I discipline my body and bring it into subjection, lest, when I have preached to others, I myself should become disqualified." You must keep your eyes fixed on the prize, remember your goal, and go through the necessary work to get there. Don't focus on your present condition, but think about where you want to be in a month, six months, or a year from now. You have to think like you are training to win your own Super Bowl.

Get Your Rest to Be Your Best

If NFL players are required to get enough rest so they can perform at their best, don't you think you need to get the right amount as well? Unfortunately, Americans today are getting less sleep than ever before. In a survey conducted in 2010 by the Centers for Disease Control and Prevention, researchers found that 30 percent of working Americans are sleeping an average of six or fewer hours per night, with night-shift workers logging even fewer winks than their daytime counterparts.[7] Today, the national average for Americans is around 6.7 hours of sleep during the weekday, down from 7 hours in 2001.[8]

I have often joked that the reason you lose weight if you sleep a lot is that you aren't up eating late at night. I have learned, however, that there is a little more going on than that. For instance, if you don't sleep, you are tired the next day; and being tired becomes an excuse for not exercising. When you are lacking in sleep, you will also be more likely to search for comfort foods that will give you quick energy to overcome the tiredness you feel. The charge you get from the high-calorie food may work for a while, but you will add unwanted pounds—much of it in that dreaded belly area. This will set the stage for obesity and even sleep apnea, which will result in more sleep loss. It's a vicious cycle that you can break only by getting enough sleep.

Dr. Michael Breus, author of *Beauty Sleep* and the clinical director of the sleep division for Arrowhead Health in Glendale, Arizona, says, "It's not so much that if you sleep, you will lose weight, but if you are sleep-deprived, meaning that you are not getting enough minutes of good quality sleep, your metabolism will not function properly."[9] He believes that the average adult needs seven-and-a-half hours of sleep at night, though some would say even that is not enough.

In a small study led by Orfeu Buxton, assistant professor at Harvard Medical School and an associate neuroscientist at Brigham and Women's Hospital in Boston, researchers controlled the sleep, diet and activities of 21 participants for five weeks to mimic the sleep patterns of shift workers. "We saw an 8 percent reduction in resting metabolic rate, or the amount of calories you burn to maintain body weight while you rest," he says. "This equates to a potential of 10 pounds of weight gain in a year, with diet and exercise remaining the same."[10] Buxton's team also found a connection between lack of sleep, interrupted sleep and a slide toward pre-diabetes. Three weeks into his study, he discovered that his subjects' pancreases had stopped responding to meals normally and began making a third less insulin. Insulin is the hormone that converts sugar to energy, and without it sugar levels rise—the hallmark of diabetes.

The two hormones that are key to sleep and weight loss are *ghrelin* and *leptin*. "Ghrelin is the 'go' hormone that tells you when to eat, and when you are sleep-deprived, you have more ghrelin," Dr. Breus explains. "Leptin is the hormone that tells you to stop eating, and when you are sleep deprived, you have less leptin."[11] In other words, if you have more ghrelin and less leptin, you will gain weight.

In another study published in 2010 in the *Annals of Internal Medicine*, researchers found that dieters who got a full night's sleep lost the same amount of weight as when they slept less. However, when those dieters got enough sleep, more than half of the weight they lost was fat, as compared to only one-fourth of their weight loss from fat when they cut back on their sleep. "If your goal is to lose fat, skipping sleep is like poking sticks in your bicycle wheels," says Dr. Plamen Penev, director of the study. "Cutting back on sleep, a behavior that is ubiquitous in modern society, appears to compromise efforts to lose fat through dieting."[12]

Jerry Kram, medical director of the California Center for Sleep Disorders in Alameda, California, concludes that "there isn't a substitute for an adequate amount of sleep."[13] For those who have a problem getting enough sleep, he and other researchers suggest taking the following actions:

- Recognize you are sleep deprived. That's a good place to begin.

- Ditch the belief that you only need six hours sleep per night.

- Stop drinking caffeine in the afternoon. Caffeine has a half-life of three to seven hours. Even if it doesn't keep you awake, it will keep you in the lighter stages of sleep that are associated with poor sleep quality.[14]

- Get some exercise—it will improve your quality of sleep.

- Watch what you eat in the afternoon and early evening. "Eating a huge dinner . . . may make you feel drowsy, but the sleep won't necessarily take," says *TODAY* show nutrition expert Joy Bauer. "When you lie down and try to sleep, your digestion will slow down, make you feel uncomfortable, and possibly keep you awake."[15]

- If your schedule is such that you can't eat until just before bedtime, eat a few healthy snacks and then have a light meal, like a bowl of cereal.

- Turn off cell phones, TVs, laptops and other electronic devices well before bedtime to give yourself a chance to relax. These stimulate the brain, and the light they produce tell the brain that it is daytime, which will disrupt your internal clock.[16]

So, guys, you gotta get your zzzs to gain your health.

Get to the Gym

We have already talked about the importance of being disciplined in your food choices, and now it is time to start being disciplined with your body. It's time to get to the gym. You can't avoid it any longer! I know how you are feeling right now. I avoided this one as long as I could. The sad fact is that the whole time I was sitting in my recliner, slowly killing myself with food, I had a gym membership. My whole family did. I used to drive my children there and drop them off so they could go in and work out and play basketball, but I never went in myself. How crazy is that?

After I finally made the decision to go into the gym and actually work out, a whole host of emotions flooded my mind. When I got on those machines, I quickly sobered at the reality of just how out of shape I was. I could only do about five minutes on the treadmill. Me, the college athlete who used to run for hours, could only walk for *five minutes*—after which time I thought I was going to die! I was frustrated, depressed and embarrassed, all at the same time.

Evidently, Satan came with me to the gym, because he whispered in my ear, "People are looking at you. They think you are pathetic. They think you are less of man because of the way you look." I was so discouraged that I almost didn't go back. But then I remembered Paul's words 1 Corinthians 9:27 that I needed to discipline my body and bring it into subjection. That meant I had to go back and try again. So I did, and each time I returned I was able to do a little bit more.

Then one day it hit me—nobody was looking at me! They were too busy looking in the mirrors at themselves to worry about what I was doing or what I looked like. To think that I almost let what I believed others were thinking about me to divert me from the goal at hand. It had all been a lie from the devil. You may also be feeling intimidated or insecure about going to the gym. But all you need is a little help with the basics, and you'll be off and running on that treadmill.

Kick-Start Exercise

Matt Fitzgerald, fitness expert and author of *Brain Training for Runners,* wrote a short article on what he calls the "Fitness ABCs." He suggests the following to help you kick-start your exercise routine:

A *Acquire some basic skills.* Ask a personal trainer at the gym to show you how to use the equipment properly, and work out with a video or with a trainer to learn how to do resistance exercises correctly. Consider purchasing a few sessions with a trainer to maximize your workout and avoid injury, or join a small group that works with a trainer.

B *Balance your routine.* Do different kinds of exercises to work out different areas of your body. Aerobic exercises will rid the body of fat and strengthen the cardiovascular and metabolic system. Strength training will help you do daily activities such as lifting objects and climbing stairs. Stretching can improve your posture and joint health and keep you from injury. Varying your routine will also help you not to tax and overuse certain muscle groups.

C *Challenge yourself.* Don't plod along. Work hard. Push yourself to go just a little faster and a little farther each time. As one fitness expert states, "If you go through the motions in the gym, you're going to get the same kind of results you get from going through the motions in a job."[17]

Maybe you don't have a gym nearby, or perhaps other factors such as cost are keeping you from exercising. If so, start walking. It's a free exercise, and it can be done with a friend, your children, a spouse and anyone else. Put on some earphones and listen to music, a speech or sermon while you walk—or even learn a new language! Take along your dog on the walk and kill two birds with one stone. Carry weights or use hiking poles to exercise the upper part of your body. Join a walking club at the local mall, or just walk there in inclement weather. You can also choose to walk on a treadmill or an elliptical machine, or just march in place.

Walking is a great form of exercise, and it's a good place for you to start if you haven't been active in a long time. Here are some tips:

- Drink a big glass of water before you begin. It will hydrate your muscles.
- Choose a good pair of shoes—they're your only equipment.
- Stretch before you start, and warm up by walking slowly for a few minutes.
- Do intermittent walking—fast, then slow.
- Set a goal for how long you will walk or how far. When you have reached your goal, cool down by walking slowly until your heart rate has dropped.
- Finish by drinking another big glass of water.

At first you may only be able to walk only a short distance, but start thinking of ways you can gradually increase the amount of steps you take each day. Some men find a pedometer works well to help them keep track of their steps and help them reach a goal of 10,000 steps a day. Pedometers aren't expensive—and trust me, what they cost will be money well spent.

Even though walking may seem like a simple exercise, you'll find that when you are walking, you are working out. When I started training for our first 5K walk, I thought there was no way I could participate, let alone finish. Getting through the whole course in the beginning was challenging, but I can do it now. My next goal is to run the whole course, not walk it.

There are walking events throughout the country—there's surely one in your town—and joining such an event is a great motivator and confidence builder. Check out the web to find many great plans that are designed to get you off from the couch to finishing a 5K run. You just have to search for them. To keep yourself motivated, constantly set newer and bigger goals for yourself. Oh, and by the way . . . don't forget to celebrate when you meet your goals. Imagine the celebration you could have after you finish your first 5K!

Sweat Is Fat Crying

There is a saying that "sweat is fat crying." That's what I want you to do—make your fat cry! Start working out and sweating so that you can burn and shed that blubber. And not only does exercise cause fat to cry, but it gives you other huge benefits as well. Here are just seven benefits of regular physical activity as reported by the Mayo Clinic:

1. It controls weight.
2. It combats health conditions and diseases.
3. It improves mood.
4. It boosts energy.
5. It promotes better sleep.
6. It puts the spark back into your sex life.
7. It can be fun!

As a general goal, most experts recommend at least 30 minutes of specific activity each day. However, to lose weight, you may need to exercise more.[18]

I want you to seriously meditate on Isaiah 40:31, our key verse for this chapter: "But those who wait on the LORD shall renew their strength; they shall mount up with wings like eagles, they shall run and not be weary, they shall walk and not faint." Think about those words when you are out for a walk or running on the treadmill. The same Holy Spirit who raised Jesus from the dead is right there comforting you and encouraging you to keep moving. That's powerful! He will give you the strength you need to take care of that wonderful creation, your body.

How to Make Time for Exercise

The number one excuse I hear from people for not exercising is lack of time. Ironically, the same people who tell me they don't have enough time to exercise have plenty of time to watch TV, do social networking, play video games, or hang out with the guys. Imagine if a player were at training camp and said he didn't have time for exercise. What do you think would happen to him?

The truth is that it's not lack of time that keeps you from doing what's best for your body; it's something deeper. Perhaps you think you don't need exercise. Perhaps you are in denial about the condition of your health. Perhaps you are afraid you will embarrass yourself—or get hurt. Perhaps you don't think you are worth the effort and expense it will take to buy the equipment or join a health club to care for yourself. But consider this: will you have time later on for multiple doctors' appointments? Will you have the money later on for the expensive medications you will have to take if you don't get healthy?

If you want to exercise and get physically fit, you will do it. If you are not serious about it, you won't. It's that simple. So, if you made the decision to take your physical fitness seriously, here are a few ideas that will help you stick to your commitment:

1. Make an appointment with yourself to exercise *at least* 30 minutes each day, five times a week. Consider this appointment *sacred*—something you don't break.

2. Take a look at your schedule to determine what keeps you so busy, and then see what can be delegated to others.

3. Take advantage of the smallest amounts of time. Do a few ab crunches at your desk or stand up and do some deep knee bends.

4. Assess just how much time you are spending watching TV, and set a time limit (and maybe even a timer) for your viewing. Record favorite programs or sports events and view them after you exercise.

5. If you are watching TV, don't just sit there—do something. Keep dumbbells, resistance bands and even a jump rope nearby so you can do a few exercises during the shows. If that is too much, just do some exercises during the commercials.

6. Find an exercise routine that you enjoy, or mix up the kinds of exercise you do.

7. Walk with a friend. Opt for "social-movia" rather than social-media.

8. If you have a family, get them involved in exercise. Too many kids today struggle with obesity and low muscle tone. Hike, play soccer or touch football, shoot a few baskets, ride bikes or ask the kids what they want to do. You'll be building memories as well as muscles.

9. If you travel for business, take along your workout clothes and even a swimsuit. Most hotels have workout rooms and pools. If they don't, many accommodate guests by offering passes to a nearby gym. If all else fails, walk the hotel stairs for 20 to 30 minutes.

10. Consider making your exercise routine the first thing you do in the morning. This way, you don't have to think about it or feel guilty if something comes up that consumes your time.

11. Ride a bike to work if possible. You will get a good workout, and it will save you money on gas.

12. Do your own yardwork and maintenance. Again, this will save you money.

Make It Fun!

Guys, the bottom line is to find something you love doing that incorporates movement and exercise—and then do it! If you choose to do something you enjoy for exercise, chances are that you will keep at it. Think outside of the box. Get involved in a basketball league, go bowling, or play racquetball or even paintball. If you used to love to swim as a kid, join a local pool; or volunteer to help work with a local youth sports league in your area. I know I said earlier "no pain, no gain," but exercise really doesn't have to be a miserable experience. In fact, it can be a lot fun. So decide today to pick a few activities that you love that will help you get fit, burn calories and build strength.

Let's Get Started

Just as football players have to constantly exercise to condition their bodies, so do you. I hope that you now feel motivated to start moving your body, and that you start doing it right away. One resource that I want to give you to help you get started is from the Centers for Disease Control and Prevention, at www.cdc.gov/physicalactivity/everyone/videos. This website contains videos that explain physical activity guidelines, gives you tips on getting started, and also shows you how to properly do muscle strengthening exercises at home and in the gym. So check it out. Finally, let me leave you with these words from Winston Churchill: "Never, never, never, never give up!"[19] I know it will be tough, but I promise that all of your hard work and determination will pay off.

Scott Boyle
Says Move It!

LOST 49 POUNDS

Before	After
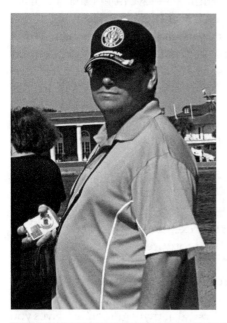	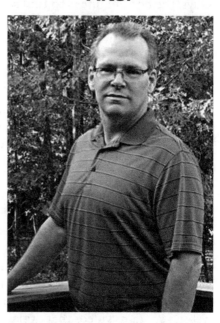

Eighteen months ago, I weighed 242 pounds and had many health issues. When I went in for my annual blood test, the results were not very encouraging—in fact, they were rather frightening. I was told that I had a buildup of plaque in my arteries, and at the time I had no idea how to get rid of it. Later on, I went in for another screening and learned that my risk factor for heart disease was 8 out of 10—with 10 being the worst it could be. My triglycerides and cholesterol were enormously high. When I learned of my condition, I decided enough is enough. I was approaching my fiftieth birthday, and I was way too young to die. We have two children and four grandkids, and I didn't want to leave them.

Two ladies in my church had started a First Place 4 Health program, so my wife and I decided to join. We made a promise to each other that no matter what happened, we would stay in the program. We started slowly. At first I did jumping jacks, bicycle crunches and half-planks. When I got so I could do these simple exercises, I began adding 30 minutes of walking, cardio exercises, and lifting dumbbells.

Today, my wife and I exercise for two hours on Saturdays and at least 30 minutes to an hour during the other days of the week. We started walking and taking our dog with us. We live on top of a hill, so when we walk down at the start of our routine, we have to come back up the hill at the end to get home. I am within 20 pounds of my weight goal according to the guidelines set for my height and age, my cholesterol counts are within normal range, and I am no longer on prescription medicine.

I have been blessed in that my wife was right with me in reaching my weight-loss goals. She has her own goals, and she's dropped four clothing sizes. We avoid going out to eat too often—we generally only go out on special occasions—and we share in the cooking and help each other eat right. We have limited going to fast-food places and have cut out fried foods. (If you really knew what was in your fast-food burger, you would change your mind about eating it. It's pretty disgusting.)

My wife and I have also stopped drinking diet soda, which causes cravings for sweets, and instead drink Red Goji tea. We also drink plenty of water. When exercising we avoid drinking Gatorade, which is loaded with sugar for energy. There are 14 grams of sugar in 8 ounces of Gatorade, and you would need to exercise a long time to burn it all off.

I have reduced my intake of sodium to almost none. Before joining First Place 4 Health, I had to take pills for acid reflux, but today I have no problems with it whatsoever. This is because I stopped eating at least three hours prior to going to bed, which prevents acid reflux from developing and gives my body a chance to burn some of the calories I took in at my last meal. I drink only two cups of coffee a day, and I add them to my fluid intake. (Regarding fluid intake, to calculate what you need each day, take your current weight and divide it in half. That answer is the number of ounces of water you should drink each day.) I also try to limit my daily sugar intake to only 15 grams, which is very hard to do.

Recently, a Tropical Café Smoothie franchise opened in our area, and we enjoy the flavorful foods and smoothies with a healthy appeal that they offer. We've also replaced eating white bread with whole-wheat bread. We now buy something called "Flatout Bread." The bread is an oval shape—flat, rather than a loaf. It is low in fat, a good source of fiber, and it is perfect for making wraps, pinwheels and a super-easy pizza. But here's the best part: it has only 90 calories.

Do you like the word *zero*? Sure you do. Well, there is a company called Walden Farms that makes some great products that have *no* calories, sugars, gluten, fat or carbs. The company sells condiments such as salad dressings, syrups, fruit spreads, BBQ sauce and pasta sauces. One other delicious and nutritious food my wife and I enjoy is a stuffed sweet potato. We cook the sweet potatoes in the microwave and then top them with ground turkey, tomato, guacamole, black olives, Greek yogurt, salsa and low-fat cheese. Sweet potatoes are low in sodium, saturated fat and cholesterol and are a good source of dietary fiber, vitamin B6, potassium, vitamin A, vitamin C and magnesium.

Let me warn you: although it is tempting to do so, don't buy into fad weight-loss programs. Remember that the extra pounds came on over time, so it will take time to get them off. Build a habit of eating healthy and exercising each day. It takes 21 days to build a habit, but you can do this. I have faith in you! And if you feel angry with yourself . . . good! Use that anger to motivate yourself to go the extra mile and spend that extra minute on the treadmill. If you are upset with yourself, you will push yourself forward.

Speaking of workouts, you don't need to be rich to exercise, nor do you have to have the most expensive equipment available. Remember Rocky Balboa in those old *Rocky* movies? Like him, you can grab a log and do lunges with it, or you can put some rocks in a wheelbarrow, deflate the tires, and push that around. You *will* get a workout.

Whatever you do, don't give up. Exercise every day. Act as if you are a contestant on *The Biggest Loser*, where no excuses are tolerated. Plan your walking time. Walk alone, or with a spouse, or with one of your children, or with a friend. Organize walks with other men who are also intent on moving their bodies.

Added weight creates costly health issues that you can avoid simply by losing the excess weight. My wife and I have found that being fit and healthy has reduced our visits to the doctors, which saves on co-pays. We require less prescription medicines, which is a definite savings that we can spend on our kids and grandkids.

You can do it! I know you can. I know you can become a healthy man of God. Remember, in Philippians 4:13 Paul states that we can do *all things* through Christ who strengthens us. Be in constant prayer to Jesus, for He is your strength, your Rock.

Man Up

Eat Up: Healthy Fats
Did you know that nuts help hinder heart attacks? According to research, one handful of raw unsalted nuts a day cuts the risk of having a heart attack in half. Healthy fats will actually help you lose fat. Your brain, skin, connective tissue and hormones all need fat, but only the good kind found in raw nuts, olives, avocado and fish. Use olive oil in recipes. Add a ¼ cup of almonds or walnuts to your salad. Mash up ¼ cup of an avocado with some chopped fresh tomatoes and a squeeze of lemon or lime for a wonderful salad dressing. Wild-caught salmon and sardines are also filled with healthy omega-3 fat.

Pump Up: Change Out that Spare Tire
Torso rotations are core-strengthening exercises that allow your torso to move through a full range of motion, targeting your back, abdominals and obliques all at once. Stand with your feet shoulder-width apart, knees slightly bent, and hold your arms out in front of your. Interlock your hands and fingers. Keeping your shoulders down, bend your elbows slightly and rotate your torso to the right until your arms are in line with your body. Rotate back through center and to the left, and continue rotating from side to side. Do about 30 of these, rest for 30 seconds, and then repeat. Do as many as you can during the day, and hold a medicine ball or dumbbell for added effort.

Reflection and Discussion Questions

1. In what ways have you allowed the American "decrease pain/increase pleasure mentality" to affect your exercise habits?

   _____

   _____

   _____

   _____

2. If Jesus visited you to discuss your health, what would He say about your current condition? What would He suggest you improve? Think about this in relationship to His words in Matthew 16:24-25.

   _____

   _____

   _____

   _____

3. Exercise is movement. What strategies can you incorporate into your daily routine to move more?

   _____

   _____

   _____

   _____

4. It is important to make a sacred appointment with yourself to exercise at least 30 minutes a day, five times per week. What is the best time for you to do this? How will you block out your calendar to make sure you do it?

   _____

   _____

   _____

   _____

5. What type of exercise do you enjoy doing? How will you incorporate this into your daily fitness routine?

_____
_____
_____
_____
_____

6. Isaiah 40:31 says that when you rely on God, He will give you the strength to walk and run. What do you need God to give you the strength to do in order to keep to your commitment to exercise each day?

_____
_____
_____
_____
_____

MY PERSONAL GAME PLAN FOR

GETTING IN SHAPE

*Beloved, I pray that you may prosper in all things
and be in health, just as your soul prospers.*

3 JOHN 2

This book is about **ACTION** and about **DOING**! In the spaces below, record what actions you are going to take to improve your health this week.

Aware—I will do the following to show I am aware of my current physical condition and that my body matters to God:

_____
_____
_____
_____
_____

Commit—I will do the following to commit to living a disciplined life and to winning over temptation:

_____
_____
_____
_____
_____
_____

Transform—This is how I will transform the way I think and live:

_____
_____
_____
_____
_____

Incorporate—I will incorporate these healthy eating habits and exercise into my daily life:

_____
_____
_____
_____
_____

Organize—This is how I will organize a team of people to help me win:

_____
_____
_____
_____
_____

Navigate—This is my action plan for healthy living and navigating my way to leaving a lasting legacy:

_____
_____
_____
_____
_____

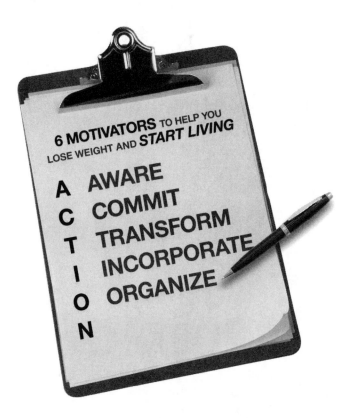

Organize

The fifth step in your journey toward getting of the couch and getting into shape is to *organize* a team of people who wan to help you win. You can't do this all on your own. You need to start building a circle of support—a team of people who will educate, encourage and equip you so you can meet your health and wellness goals. There is strength in numbers, and you will achieve more and experience greater success if you have a team of likeminded people supporting you. So choose your team wisely, and start winning together.

Chapter 9

Stronger Together

Though one may be overpowered by another, two can withstand him.
And a threefold cord is not quickly broken.
ECCLESIASTES 4:12

I've heard many women say they dread football season. It's the time of year when they feel as if they lose the men in their lives to this game—a game that many of them don't understand.

Why *are* we men so passionate about football? I mean, think about it. What happens to most of us when football season starts? From the minute the NFL starts talking about the draft, we zone in on the upcoming season . . . sometimes to the point of obsession. We get out our team jerseys. We eagerly await the new players who will be drafted to "our team." We schedule our lives around the games. We get mobile updates on our phones with the latest scores and stats so we won't miss a thing. We might forget special events, birthdays and anniversaries, but we can spout off our favorite quarterback's completion percentage, yards per completion, touchdowns, interceptions, fumbles and QBR.

Our relationship with football is deeply personal to us. It's one we have nourished and developed over a long period of time. We feel as if we know the players on our team. We form bonds with them during the season—and with the other guys who join us to watch the games. We celebrate with our players when they win, and we mourn with them when they lose. We yell and scream right along with our "teammates" when the other side (or the officials) do something we don't like. We feel our team's loss when a key player is injured and has to miss a portion of the season. Win or lose, we are die-hard fans.

We Like Teams . . . in Sports but Not in Life

Let's face it: we love teams when it comes to sports, but we don't like them when it comes to life. If we're honest with ourselves, when it comes to everyday life, we prefer to go solo. As men, we like to be independent and in charge of our own destiny. We like to do things on our own without any help. For the most part, we don't ask for directions, and we don't read them either. We aren't deeply personal, and we don't like to share too much—especially when it comes to our emotions.

We form our most intimate relationships with our wives and children, not with other men. As a result, we tend to have a much smaller network of close friends than our wives. We focus on taking care of our families and careers, not on building social networks, and zone in on fixing things instead of expressing our feelings. We really don't like to talk all that much—we could commute to work with another guy and not say a word the whole time, and everything would be just fine. If we took that same car ride with our wife, she would think we were upset at her. She would get all bent out of shape. Women need to talk. They need the closeness and intimacy they find in sharing their thoughts and feelings with another person.

Take, for instance, what happens in the women's room versus what happens in the men's room. You know what I'm talking about: those unwritten rules of bathroom behavior that your dad never sat you down and explained—the ones you just have to learn as you grow from a boy into a man. Think about it. When guys go out to a restaurant or other event, they go to the bathroom *alone*. In fact, you probably feel uncomfortable when there are other guys in there with you. You might even give a "courtesy cough" if you're in a stall to let someone who walks in know you're there.

Then, of course, there is the urinal rule. If there are three urinals and another guy is at one of them, you never, ever, use the one closest to him. You don't talk during this time, and you certainly don't make eye contact. It's just too close for comfort. In fact, the only time it is acceptable to talk to another man in the bathroom is when he is washing his hands—and then only for a quick nod and hello. There is no exchange of business cards. You focus on doing your business and get out of there as quickly as possible.

Now, I don't have any firsthand experience in this area, but it seems to me that quite the opposite occurs in the women's room. When women go to the bathroom, it turns into an event. I mean, they go in teams—in packs. And needing to go seems to be contagious. When one woman says she has to go, every woman around thinks it's a good idea as well. And they take *hours* in there. I have a wife and two daughters, so I know of what I speak. I have a *lot* of experience in waiting for them. They must talk and socialize in there, catch up on what's going on in each other's lives and re-do make-up, and I'm sure there is a lot of laughing and crying going on as well. They network, exchange contact information and forge alliances. I mean, it's a production. It's a wonder they even remember what they went in there to do.

We men are just wired differently. That's not good or bad; it's just different. And when it comes to the concept of building relationships and supporting one another, women tend to be better at it than men, especially when it comes to health, weight loss, wellness and getting in shape. Women love to talk to other women about how their diet is going, how much weight they need to lose, and what weight-loss recipes they have tried. They love to start walking groups or join aerobics or Pilates classes so they can build relationships while they exercise.

Us guys, on the other hand, have a tendency to bury our heads in chips and salsa when it comes to our health. We don't like to go to the doctor. We don't like to eat fancy soups and salads. We don't want to find three other guys whom we can walk around the block with a thousand times as we talk about what's happening on some popular TV show, or how our wives are never home on time for dinner, or what we are going to wear out on our date the following night. Yet even though we are wired differently than women, we have to start developing an appreciation of women's ability to find a network of people who can come alongside them and help them get back in the game of living life and winning again. We have to come to the point where we realize we can't do this alone. It's going to take a team of people to follow through with our commitment to get off the couch and get into shape.

Why do we need a team? Walter Payton, Hall of Fame running back for the Chicago Bears, hit the nail on the head when he said, "We are stronger together than we are alone." We will win more, achieve more and succeed more when we work together with others to reach a common goal. We have to let go of the Rambo philosophy of life—the idea that we can conquer it all alone by taking out every obstacle in our path and winning every fight by ourselves.

I know what you're thinking right now. This is a hard one. You are probably saying to yourself, *But he doesn't know me. He doesn't know what I can do, and that I can do this alone.* Trust me on this one, and keep reading, because in this chapter I'm going to tell you exactly why you need a team to help you win in the area of your health. Once again, we will start with what our Playbook, the Bible, says about this idea.

There's Strength in Numbers

Why do you need a team? What's the value in it? What will it do for you? Well, the Bible answers these questions for you in Ecclesiastes 4:9-12, which says:

> Two are better than one, because they have a good reward for their labor. For if they fall, one will lift up his companion. But woe to him who is alone when he falls, for he has no one to help him up. Again, if two lie down together, they will keep warm; but how can one be warm alone? Though one may be overpowered by another, two can withstand him. And a threefold cord is not quickly broken.

This is an important biblical principle, and one that will have a huge impact on your life. It's the principle that *two are better than one*. Two can withstand the enemy; so, if you want to be strong, find a partner to act as the third cord of a strand. You were never meant to do life alone. In fact, way back in the beginning when God created the world and everything in it—right after He made Adam and placed him in the Garden of Eden to live—we hear God say for the first time that something isn't good: "It is not good that man should be alone" (Genesis 2:18). It was part of God's plan for you to have people with you for help and support—people to do life with.

Teamwork is mentioned throughout the Bible, where it is used as a model for successful Christian living. One of the reasons why God created the institution of marriage—and why Christ taught so much about the Body of believers—is because teams are needed to promote the gospel. Each person plays an integral role and is needed for the whole Body to function (see 1 Corinthians 12:12-17). During the Early Church era, teams were used for discipleship and in the spreading of the gospel. Teams were the way Christ intended the Church to operate. There were to be teams of Christlike people, each working together to use their God-given strengths and abilities to fulfill the Great Commission of reaching the entire world with the gospel. God's plan has always involved teamwork. Why? Because teamwork produces mutual success, provides mutual support, and builds mutual strength.

Teamwork Produces Mutual Success

When we read about having a "good reward of their labor" in Ecclesiastes 4:9, it is emphasizing the mutual success that comes through teamwork. Teaming up with people who share your goals will help you to experience success in life. Why do you think Satan wants to isolate you? He knows that if he can keep you alone instead of with people who will push you to make positive changes in your life, he can keep you in bondage. He can keep you from winning. Satan has a divide-and-conquer strategy because he knows there is strength in numbers.

If you are going to experience the reward of a better body and a better lifestyle, you have to be part of a team. You have to come to the point where you are willing to say, "You know what? I need help." In the beginning it might be only one trusted friend to whom you can turn, but you have to go to *somebody* and admit you need help.

Teamwork Provides Mutual Support

Having a team around you will also provide you with mutual support. In Ecclesiastes 4:10 we read, "For if they fall, one will lift up his companion. But woe to him who is alone when he falls. For he has no one to help him up." What a sad statement—"he has no one to help him up." When you do life alone, there won't be anybody there to help you when you fall. There won't be anybody there to support you. That is why you need a team. When you give in to temptation or slip back into those bad habits, the people on your team will be right there waiting to help get you back on track, and they will encourage you to keep pressing forward.

Think about what happens in a race. When you run alongside some-one, you push each other to do your best and run faster. When fatigue sets in and you want to quit or you are tempted to just walk, your partner keeps you moving. Teammates are your cheerleaders who keep you focusing on crossing that finish line. You need these people around you when times get hard and you are weak and tired.

Teamwork Builds Mutual Strength

Finally, having a team builds mutual strength. We see this in Ecclesiastes 4:12 where it says, "Two can withstand him, and a threefold cord is not quickly broken." Two is great, for sure, but when you add that third per-son, you're even stronger. It is not easy to break a threefold (three-strand) cord. A team of 5 to 10 people means you have more people praying for you, more people speaking wisdom into your life, more people providing you with wise counsel, and more people encouraging you. Trust me, guys, life change happens best through a team. Together, you will be stronger.

The Spirit of Pride

Now, it seems quite obvious that there are many benefits of joining a team. So what keeps us from doing it? Why is it so difficult for us? It is the attitude that we can do it alone, and that attitude is birthed out of one thing: pride.

Satan is proud. He revolted against God when he said, "I will ascend to heaven. I will exalt my throne above the stars of God . . . I will be like the Most High" (Isaiah 14:13-14). "I will . . . I will . . . I will . . ." Do you find yourself making these types of statements? "I will eat whatever I want. I will sit right here as long as I want. I will be just fine." This spirit is contrary to God's will and plan for your life. This spirit of rebellion and pride is what led Satan to fall from the position of being a glorious angel in heaven to becoming God's adversary. Satan wants to plant that same spirit in you in order to isolate you.

Proverbs 16:18 says, "Pride goes before destruction, and a haughty spirit before a fall." I've said it before, and I'll say it again: Satan wants to kill you. He wants to destroy you, and the tool he is going to use is your pride to keep you from building a circle of support. He does not want a team of people around you who will help keep you focused on honoring God with your life and your body. So it's time to recognize that you can't make the changes you need to make unless you let go of your pride. You need to face the fact that you can't do this alone and start thinking about getting a good team of people around you to help you win.

Let's take a look at an example from the life of Moses, a mighty man in the Bible, who had to learn this lesson the hard way. Yes, even Moses had to come to the realization that he needed a team. And it took a good "man-to-man" talk with his father-in-law, Jethro, to set him straight.

Check Up

Big Belly = Difficulty Breathing

Recent medical research shows that obesity increases the risk of asthma and other breathing problems. In one study, obese individuals comprised 75 percent of all emergency department visits for asthma. The changes in the body's shape that occur in overweight individuals are detrimental to breathing—the excess weight pushes the lungs upward and restricts chest motion, which results in under-expanded lungs, shallower breaths, increased inflammation and narrowing of the airways. From a physiological standpoint, this alters the airflow, respiratory compliance, lung volumes, peripheral airway diameter and airway hyper-responsiveness. These mechanical effects also rob the body and tissues of oxygen, resulting in shortness of breath, weakness and easy fatigability. Sometimes, full-time oxygen (with a cumbersome oxygen tank) is required to treat this condition. Weight loss has been shown to lead to improved breathing, lung function and physiologic parameters.[1]

Moses' Man-to-Man Talk

Moses was an amazing dude who accomplished many extraordinary things during his lifetime. Yet there are several examples in the Bible where Moses had to ask for help—times when he just couldn't win by himself. For instance, he asked for help when God first called him. He told God that he didn't feel he could go to Pharaoh alone, because he couldn't speak plainly. So God gave him his brother, Aaron, to do the talking for him (see Exodus 3).

Another time, the Israelites were in a battle with the Amalekites, and whenever Moses' arms dropped to his sides, the battle went against them. He didn't have the strength and stamina to hold up his arms for the amount of time needed to defeat the opposition, so he had to bring two other men, Joshua and Hur, to help him. They held up Moses' arms while the battle raged below them, and eventually the Israelites won.

There is one other notable story of Moses not being able to handle something on his own—an instance when he needed help and direction. The story is told in Exodus 18. Moses, at God's instruction, had taken a bunch of slaves out to the desert and was leading them on a hike to a place called the "Promised Land." Believe me, things didn't go well. The ex-slaves were not used to making decisions, because a slave boss had always told them what to do and when to do it. They were not used to getting along with each other without an overseer forcing them to comply with certain rules. What Moses had on his hands was a personnel nightmare and a judicial headache.

One day, Moses' father-in-law, Jethro, came to the camp of the Israelites along with his daughter, Zipporah (Moses' wife), and their two sons. Moses went down to meet them. They greeted one another, and Moses began to tell his father-in-law all about the good things God was doing for Israel.

"That's wonderful," Jethro told his son-in-law. "Praise be to God for rescuing you from the Egyptians and Pharaoh."

Moses then told his father-in-law about some of the hardships they had encountered and how God had saved them. Again, Jethro was delighted at the goodness of God toward the people. After a while, Aaron and the elders of Israel came to supper, and after a pleasant evening they all went to bed.

The next morning, Moses took his seat to act as judge for the people. The crowd stood around him from morning to night, debating and asking questions. Jethro stood nearby and watched all of what was going on. That evening he said to Moses, "What are you doing for the people?

Why are you sitting alone as the judge while all these people stand around you from sunup to sundown?"

"Well, the people come to me to seek God's will," Moses replied. "Whenever they have a dispute, they bring it to me, and I decide between the two parties. I inform them of God's laws and decrees."

"Ah, Moses," said Jethro. "What you are doing is not good. You are only going to wear yourself out, and the people right along with you. The work is too heavy for you, and you can't handle it alone. So listen. You must be the peoples' representative before God and bring their disputes to Him. Teach them the laws and decrees, and show them the way to live and the duties they are to perform. Okay?"

"But . . . but . . ." Moses began.

"Wait, I'm not finished," said Jethro. "Select capable men—a team—from among the people. Choose men who fear God and who hate dishonesty. Appoint them to serve as officials over groups of 1,000, 100, 50 and 10. Let them serve as judges for the people at all times. Let them decide the simple cases on their own. Allow them to decide which cases should come to you for a decision."

"Oh!" Moses said as the light began to dawn on him. He now saw that there was a different way to manage God's people.

"If you will do this your load will be lighter," said Jethro, "because the men you appoint will share the burden with you. In this way, the people will be satisfied, and you will be able to stand the strain of the work."

Now, the Bible leaves out a lot of the little details in this story. Why did Jethro come to Moses with his wife and two sons? Maybe Jethro's daughter put him up to going to Moses and having that father-in-law to son-in-law talk. If Moses was spending all day long judging the people from sunup to sundown, he probably wasn't spending much time at home with his wife and kids. The job was too much for him, and it is quite possible that other things were starting to suffer in Moses' life—such as his relationships. After all, Jethro said that what he was doing *wasn't good.*

Moses needed another man to come alongside him and show him a better way to live—a better way to handle a difficult situation. The solution to the problem was to form a team of people to help him. Thankfully for all involved, Moses listened. He heeded this wise advice from his father-in-law and put the plan into action.

Jethro must have felt confident that things were going to get better, because the Bible says he left and returned to his home, and there is no mention of him taking Zipporah and the boys with him. They stayed with Moses. The plan must have worked, because Moses lived to be 120 years old. When he died, his eyes were not weak, and his strength was not gone (see Deuteronomy 34:7). He was in great shape even at the age of 120! Perhaps the reason was because he had moved from living an isolated life to living a supported life. He moved from doing life alone to building a team around him.

Moving from Isolated to Supported

Let's carefully examine the series of steps that Moses had to go through to learn this important lesson about the value of a team.

Step 1: Recognize the Problem

Moses was trying to go it alone, and he needed to recognize that he had a problem. He probably didn't know what to do in this situation, and it likely seemed insurmountable to him. The weight of the responsibility was wearing him out. You might feel the same way right now; as if there is no hope for your health situation. You may feel it's too big an obstacle to tackle or overcome. No one—not even Moses—can go through life alone. The Bible says that in the multitude of counsel there is safety and wisdom (see Proverbs 11:14). Moses had spent many years going it alone and was used to doing it all, but that didn't mean it was what was best for him or for the people. He needed to recognize that he needed help.

Step 2: Face Reality

Perhaps Moses was a little taken aback when, after he had bragged to his father-in-law about all he and God had done, Jethro came on with a rather strong criticism of his leadership style and how he was managing his life. Moses thought he was doing great all by himself, and he thought he was doing what God told him to do. Maybe Moses' face flushed with a little bit of anger. Maybe he bit his tongue to keep from saying what he was really thinking. But somewhere along the way, he decided to listen to Jethro, and he realized that his father-in-law might be right.

Okay, guys, here it is; a valuable lesson that we all can learn as well. Moses was teachable! He listened to instruction. When another man said that something he was doing was not good, Moses heard him. In the same way, you need to listen to wise counsel—the kind of counsel you will find within a group of people who care about you. Be like Moses and get a team of people who will help you deal with your health issues. Then listen to them—especially if they have been there, done that.

You will go further in achieving your weight loss and fitness goals when you have a team of men to speak wisdom into your life and help you through the rough times. So take a look at your situation. Are you trying to go it alone? Should you be? Would a team of dedicated Christians strengthen you? Is it time you faced the reality of your situation and came to the conclusion that you don't have everything under control?

Step 3: Find a Team

Moses knew the Law of God very well, and he was uniquely qualified for his work. Yet, in taking on all the responsibility, he had submitted himself to a life-crushing burden. He needed to find the right people to help him accomplish the task of keeping order. The same goes for you. When you have the right team in place, they will be there to help you reach our goals and still be in one piece at the end of it.

Pick your teammates carefully. Jethro told Moses to select men who were up to the task—not lazy men (see Exodus 18:21). Only particular men were fit for the job Moses needed done. They were to be:

- "Able men": men of ability
- "Such as fear God": men of godliness
- "Men of truth": men of God's Word
- "Hating covetousness": men of honor

These are the types of teammates you need to be looking for as well; men who have the ability to help you, who love God, who are grounded in God's Word, and who have integrity and honor.

Step 4: Take Action

Things got better for Moses once he listened to Jethro's suggestions and followed his advice. Soon, Jethro departed and left Moses with a new perspective. The lesson for us is that we need a team around us because the losing-weight-and-get-healthy journey is tough. Moses had to personally commit to change and how he lived his life. He had to set new goals for his health so he would not wear out. He had to learn to enjoy his journey with the Lord, and he had to learn that the task was not all on him. Once he became teachable and gathered the right people around him, I'm sure his stress level decreased. Things probably started to flourish, and life likely settled down into a more orderly routine. The same thing is possible for us—we just have to get the right people around us so we can flourish. We have to listen and learn like our mighty man Moses.

Teamwork Works

If you want to lose weight, join a team—preferably a competing team. In a recent study conducted as part of the 2009 Shape Up Rhode Island campaign, a group of 3,300 overweight or obese participants with a BMI of 31.2 or greater were placed into teams of 5 to 11 members. The participants were told that they would be competing as a team in three areas: weight loss, physical activity, and the number of steps they took each day as measured by a pedometer. Interestingly, team members recorded their weight and activity via an online tracking system, and they received feedback online from other members about their personal and team goals. It was a kind of virtual competition.

Researchers found that those who shed at least 5 percent of their initial body weight during the competition were likely to be on the same teams. Furthermore, those who had a higher level of social influence with their teammates increased their weight loss by *20 percent*, with team captains losing more weight than other participants. The study also revealed that couples who attempted to lose weight together did better than when one of them tried to go it alone.

"People around us affect our health behaviors," said Tricia Leahey, a lead researcher on the study. "It could be quite beneficial if a bunch of friends that choose to lose weight make healthy food choices together, and hold each other accountable to those choices." She adds, "We know that obesity can be socially contagious, but now we know that social networks play a significant role in weight loss as well, particularly team-based weight-loss competitions. . . . Being surrounded by others with similar healthy goals all working to achieve the same thing [can really help our] weight-loss efforts."[2]

Start Thinking About the Draft

Just like the teams in the pros, you need to start thinking about who you are going to draft to be on your team. It's not an option—you have to get a good team to support you on this journey of getting in shape. It's time to do the research and start scouting so you can choose your teammates wisely. It's time to get *organized*.

Once again, the bottom line is that when you are alone, you will not be as strong as when you join with others. You need other people when it comes to honoring God with your body and leading a healthy lifestyle. In the next chapter we will discuss how to form your team in more depth, but for now, just remember (and keep telling yourself) that together you are stronger.

Steve Fruit
No Longer a Loner

LOST 29 POUNDS

Before	After
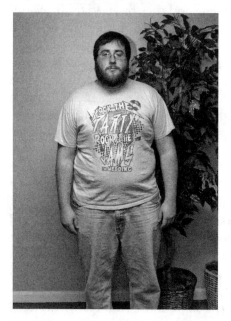	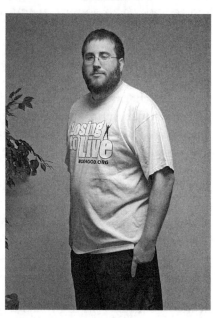

I am 26 years old. In school, I had always been overweight and, overall, larger than my friends. I had little money while I was in college, so I ate at McDonald's because I could get the most food for the least price. I drank huge sodas, because at one place I could get gargantuan drinks for little money. I also ate lots of high-sodium Ramen noodles and other typical college food.

I have known Steve Reynolds for years, and I knew he lost a lot of weight and started a program called the Losing to Live weight-loss competition. He invited me to attend several times through Facebook, but I always put it off. I would use excuses like, "I'm too busy with classes," or, "It's not that bad; I can lose weight at any time."

After graduating from college, I began to look for a job to start my career. It was then I realized I needed to do something about my weight, because it wasn't happening. So I joined the Losing to Live competition. When I weighed in for the first time, I weighed 299 pounds. I was shocked. I didn't know my weight had been creeping up that much.

Like most young people, I hadn't had the health scares that older obese people have to warn them, so I was unaware my health and wellbeing was in jeopardy. Like most people my age, I didn't know that if I was overweight and had an accident that required surgery, I would be in trouble. Surgery success rates on obese people are not good, and surgeons really don't like to operate on fat people.

During that first competition, I ended up losing 29 pounds. I decided not to join the next competition because of my work schedule, but I kept doing the program on my own, and I lost another 5 to 10 pounds. But, over time, I began to go back to my old ways, and slowly the weight crept back on. A year later, I decided I had better get back into the competition, and now my weight is back down to what it was when I quit.

I'm shy and a tad apprehensive when entering into a new situation, so I wasn't sure about being on a team. But I really like the team atmosphere at the competition. If I gained weight one week, my team members would say, "That's all right," and they would encourage me to continue on. People of all different ages and walks of life participated, and there was a flood of information from the leaders and everyone in the class. The whole competition is about eating and moving. This was not a new idea for me, but being with a group of 10 people whom I didn't want to let down was. Being engaged for 12 weeks also helped, as did being in a competition to beat the other teams. It all worked together.

I know a guy who is 20 to 30 pounds overweight. He's from a culture that pushes food at people. I told him, "I know you don't want to offend anyone, but you don't have to eat so much. Just eat less." Of course, once in a while most of us overeat, so I always tell people that if they overeat one day, just cut back the next. I also like to encourage people that, no matter what age they are, they need to get active—to start moving.

I also advise people to start exercising. My grandmother was overweight and died due to complications of diabetes. My grandfather, on the other hand, walks every day. At the age of 85 now, he is still in great shape. Truthfully, our household didn't eat too badly, but my problem was that I didn't exercise. I just laid around. That went on for years. Since I have a big build, I just accepted that I was going to be big, and I didn't do anything about my weight.

Even though I didn't want to exercise, I started doing so. In the beginning, I began too fast and hard, and I made myself sick. So my advice is to start slowly—maybe only five minutes a day at first. Later on, when you are stronger, you can extend your time. Find a friend to go with you to the gym. That person doesn't have to be at your exercise level. If he or she is working out at a higher level than you are, it's all right. You still have support in your new effort. There's no way around it—you have to both eat less and exercise more. Our first team walked/ran the 5K every Sunday before the meeting. I walked mostly because I wanted to support my leader. When it came to the actual 5K, I was able to sprint a little.

Each time I'm in a competition, I find a way to cut back a little more. This time, I have been going out to eat with friends. That doesn't sound like cutting back, but then, the next couple of days after eating out, I cut back. I've also learned to make substitutions in my diet. I discovered whole-grain pasta, and it tastes just as good to me as regular pasta, and it is more nutritious. I love coconut macaroons, and I found a low-calorie macaroon. One macaroon is only 15 calories, and it is a satisfying treat. It's worth your time to spend a couple of minutes on the Internet looking for alternatives to what you have been eating.

My biggest advice is to stay motivated and don't try to do too much at the beginning. Join a team of people who will support you and take small steps, and soon you will get where you want to be with your health.

Man Up

Eat Up: Keep Your Arteries Clear

You fry, you die! Frying at high temperatures has been shown to increase the risk of cancer, so get rid of the grease and bake, boil or sauté instead. Avoid the harmful saturated fats found in animal products and dairy, because they clog your arteries and raise your triglyceride levels and your LDL (bad) cholesterol levels. As we mentioned in a previous chapter, trans fats are even more dangerous because they raise bad cholesterol levels while lowering good cholesterol levels, so especially try to avoid these. You can do this by avoiding processed foods, which almost always contain trans fats. Also, remember that while the label may say "no trans fats," the law allows manufacturers to add one-half a serving without disclosing it. Go to the ingredient list and search for any hydrogenated or partially hydrogenated oil. If that ingredient is listed, the product contains trans fats.

Pump Up: Get-Off-the-Wall Triceps Press

Give your triceps a burn by doing this simple exercise. Start out by facing a wall. Position your hands on the wall shoulder-width apart, and place your feet on the floor, also shoulder-width apart. Lean forward to a 45-degree angle and do a push-up by lowering yourself forward until your nose touches the wall. Then push away from the wall back to your starting position. For a deeper muscle burn, spread your fingers apart and push off your fingertips. Do as many reps as you can, rest, and then repeat.

Reflection and Discussion Questions

1. Men tend to like teams in sports, but not in life. Why do you think men like to go it alone?

   _____

   _____

   _____

   _____

2. After reading this chapter, what are some of the benefits of working with others in your efforts to lead a healthier lifestyle?

   _____

   _____

   _____

   _____

   _____

3. In this chapter, we discussed the man-to-man talk that Jethro had with Moses, his son-in-saw. What stood out to you the most about this conversation?

   _____

   _____

   _____

   _____

4. Are you currently living an isolated or a supported lifestyle? If you are isolated, what steps will you take to seek support from others?

   _____

   _____

   _____

   _____

   _____

5. How would you describe the perfect team member to help you on your journey? How will you recognize this perfect weight-loss partner when he appears?

_____

_____

_____

_____

_____

6. Ecclesiastes 4:12 says, "A threefold cord is not quickly broken." What will be your first step in putting together a strong team?

_____

_____

_____

_____

_____

MY PERSONAL GAME PLAN FOR

GETTING IN SHAPE

*Beloved, I pray that you may prosper in all things
and be in health, just as your soul prospers.*
3 JOHN 2

This book is about **ACTION** and about **DOING**! In the spaces below, record what actions you are going to take to improve your health this week.

Aware—I will do the following to show I am aware of my current physical condition and that my body matters to God:

_____
_____
_____
_____
_____

Commit—I will do the following to commit to living a disciplined life and to winning over temptation:

_____
_____
_____
_____
_____
_____

Transform—This is how I will transform the way I think and live:

_____
_____
_____
_____

Incorporate—I will incorporate these healthy eating habits and exercise into my daily life:

_____

_____

_____

_____

_____

Organize—This is how I will organize a team of people to help me win:

_____

_____

_____

_____

_____

Navigate—This is my action plan for healthy living and navigating my way to leaving a lasting legacy:

_____

_____

_____

_____

_____

Chapter 10

Drafting Your Team

As iron sharpens iron, so a man sharpens the countenance of his friend.
PROVERBS 27:17

"I don't need 5,000 fans. I just need a few good friends." This Facebook post recently caught my attention with its powerful message. It's so true. When it comes to life and friendship, quality is better than quantity. Let's face it: how many friends do you still have from high school or college? Probably not many.

However, those close relationships you do have that stem from your youth likely represent lifelong bonds. They are the people whom, when you look back on your life, you can't imagine not being there. They laughed with you and rejoiced during the good times, and they were there to pull you up and help you stand strong during the rough times. They lived life with you.

It's that way with me and some of the guys with whom I played football. We started out as teammates for the game, but through the years we've become teammates for life. Remember back in chapter 1 when I talked about my buddy Roy Jones, and how we pushed each other to be the best in football? Well, after 34 years, he is still one of my closest friends.

We met on the football field at Liberty. I will never forget the first time I saw him when I ran onto the practice field. There was this stumpy, hotheaded lineman shouting my name as he stood over a 12-inch-wide, 8-foot long-board used for our board drills. Roy was an inner-city kid from Cincinnati, Ohio, and he wanted my job on the field. We were as different as night is from day, and we probably wouldn't have become so close if we hadn't been forced to interact with one another on the field.

Our coach, Lee Kaltenback, had a tradition. If you could drive-block the starter off the board, his job was yours for the day; but if you got beat on the board drill three days in a row, you lost your starting job for the week. This was all the motivation Roy needed. He wasn't even six feet tall, but he was mean as snot and had no front teeth. He even looked intimidating, and I was his target. His dad owned a bar back in "Cincy," as he called it, and he had been in more bar fights than I could count. So, as you can imagine, we went at it many times.

Remember that I said he pushed me—and I pushed him, literally. The fact is that I grew to look forward to hearing him shout, "Where is Steve

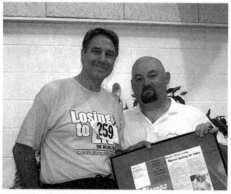

Reynolds?" Our battles were classic and memorable, and usually the rest of the team would circle around us to watch.

We sharpened one another. All of those scuffles and brawls on the field helped hone our skills for battle with our opponents during our games. While we did not become friends right away, God used that time of competition in a way that pulled us together for a lifetime. Being on the field with Roy meant a lot to me, especially since I knew he pushed me on the practice field to be a much better player.

After we left Liberty, Roy played an integral part in helping me start my ministry in northern Virginia. To this day, we still communicate often with each other. He is more than just a former football teammate; he is a cherished friend—one who has played a huge role in whom I have become. He is a valued member of my team for life.

As Proverbs 27:17 says, "As iron sharpens iron, so a man sharpens the countenance of his friend." When you interact with others, they sharpen you, and you sharpen them. If you are going to start changing how you live, you have to learn how to get this principle working in your favor. It is so important to understand that no matter who you are, the people around you have an impact on you.

The question is *how* these people will have an impact on you. Will they impact you in a positive way and make you better? Or will they impact you in a negative way and keep you from achieving all that you were meant to do? This chapter is all about finding those people who are going to push you to be better than you think you can be, just like Roy pushed me on the football field. You need to find people who will help you get off that couch and change the way you look and feel.

When I laid claim to putting this principle to work in my life—of finding people who would sharpen me—something really cool I had never noticed before jumped out at me from this verse in Proverbs: the word "countenance." When I looked up this word in the original Hebrew (*panim*), I found it means "face." It literally means the face or surface—the presence of a person, or how you present yourself. I had to start looking for people to bring into my life who would sharpen my countenance and not only help me live a godly life but also help me change how I presented myself.

I needed to start drafting people to be on my health and wellness team so I could start winning again and get back into the game of life. I needed a good push to get up and get moving, and I needed to bring people around me who would push me to try harder and continue going. I had to start thinking about drafting my team. But the question of whom I should pick loomed in my mind. I had to have a plan that would help me choose my teammates wisely, and I needed to think about how I could get the people who were already on my life team to move with me in my new direction toward my new goal. I knew this wasn't going to be an easy task, but I was confident it would pay off in the end if I did it correctly.

This was a crucial step and a pivotal point in my journey. Therefore, it was imperative that the first person who I asked to help me—my first draft pick—was God. I figured if I started with Him and let Him guide me in these crucial decisions, everything else would fall into place.

God . . . Your First Draft Pick

In the same way, the first thing you need to do when thinking about the draft picks for your team is to look to God to be number one. It all starts with Him. You are never going to succeed in this journey of getting into shape without having God on your team. He is the creator and sustainer of all life, and He needs to be your Coach, your guide and your source of strength.

Proverbs 24:10 says, "If you faint in the day of adversity, your strength is small." If you try to do this all on your own, chances are you are going to "faint" or fail. Why? Because on your own your strength is small, but with God, all things are possible (see Matthew 19:26)! You need to tap into His extraordinary power. His strength will keep you going, help you overcome all the hurdles and obstacles that Satan throws in your direction, and enable you to win.

First, however, you have to plug yourself into that power source. Just think about that treadmill sitting in your basement or in your room collecting dust—the one you use as a place to throw your clothes. It isn't going to do you any good until you plug it in, turn it on, and actually start walking on it. It's the same way with God. You have to plug into His power source and set your mind on doing things His way. You do this by praying and asking Him to be your Coach and to start guiding your steps as you begin to honor Him with your body and how you live your life.

John 3:16 gives us the game plan for making this happen: "For God so loved the world that He gave His only begotten Son, that whoever believes in Him should not perish but have everlasting life." Perhaps you have heard of this famous Bible verse. It is often displayed on banners and posters at sporting events. Tim Tebow actually wore it on his eye paint during the 2009 BCS championship game. As a result, an incredible 92 million people searched "John 3:16" on Google during or shortly after the game!

You need to know that God loves you so much and desires an awesome relationship with you. He is the source of abundant life on earth and eternal life in heaven, and He wants to provide this to you. The problem is that God is holy, and you, like all people, are unholy. You have broken God's laws, which the Bible calls "sin," and the penalty is eternal death and hell.

The good news is that God will forgive you for whatever you have done. He makes this forgiveness available through Jesus Christ, His sinless Son, who came to earth, died on the cross as payment for your sin, was buried and rose victoriously from the grave. To be forgiven and receive eternal life, you must believe in Jesus Christ as your Savior and Lord (see Acts 16:31). This requires turning from your sin and putting your trust in Jesus as the one and only way to heaven (see John 14:6).

Now, please understand that God is a perfect gentleman. He will not just barge into your life, but He will gladly join you if you invite Him. The following is an invitation prayer to make this commitment:

Dear God, I'm a sinner. Because of my sin, I deserve to spend eternity in hell. I believe Jesus died on the cross, was buried and rose from the grave for my sins. I turn from my sins and put my faith in Jesus Christ. Thank You for saving me today, and help me to serve You the rest of my life. In Jesus' name I pray. Amen.

The next thing you want to do is develop your relationship with God and make it stronger and stronger. Reading the Bible, spending time in prayer and attending a good church are just a few ways to strengthen your walk.

I love the word picture Jesus used in John 15:5 when He said, "I am the vine, you are the branches. He who abides in Me, and I in him, bears much fruit; for without Me you can do nothing." What happens when a branch gets disconnected from the vine? It withers and dies. Jesus is the vine, and you and I are just the branches. If you stay closely connected to Christ and abide in Him, He will be with you and will help you do what seems to be impossible. You will bear much fruit.

With the help of your heavenly Father, your Coach, you will be able to overcome the sin in your life that is keeping you on the couch. You will be able to overcome emotional eating. You will be able to overcome addictions and laziness. You will be able to counteract the lies that Satan throws at you with the truth from God's Word. So make God your Coach and start following His game plan.

Negotiating Negativity

When it comes to examining who is on your team, one of the most difficult steps is dealing with the negative people around you who are negatively impacting your life. In 1 Corinthians 15:33, Paul says, "Do not be deceived: 'Evil company corrupts good habits.' " If you hang out with evil people, they will corrupt your good habits. My point is this: if you are going to win, you must deal with the negative people you may already have on your team.

In my own life, I actually had to start with my mother. I live 180 miles from her, so it's not like she was feeding me every day, but I didn't get to be 100 pounds in the first grade without my parents feeding me and having an impact on me. My mother expresses her love through food, which is typical of a "Southern Momma," and that food included lots of grease, sugar and calories. So when I decided I was going to lose 100 pounds—when that goal became my focus—I had to sit down and have a heart-to-heart with my mom. I was pretty direct with her. The conversation went like this:

Mom, Papa (my grandfather) died of diabetes, and now you have diabetes. We seem to all be dealing with this horrible disease, and I don't want to die from it. I believe it is very possible that if I lose weight, I can lose the diabetes. If I can get rid of this by losing weight, I am going to do it. Mom, something has got to change. I have to do things differently, and I need your support.

This wasn't an easy conversation to have. I love my mom and didn't want to hurt her, but I knew it was the right thing to do. It was the best thing for our whole family. The incredible thing was that, thankfully, God began working in her life, and today she has lost lots of weight herself. Every Wednesday night at Thomas Road Baptist Church in Lynchburg, Virginia, Alfred and Betsy Reynolds, my parents, sit down with a team in the Losing to Live competition at their church. I had to go to my own mom and say, "Mom, I need you on my team. I need your help to change. I want to help you change, too—to change for the better." I will never regret having this pivotal conversation.

The fact is that you may have to do the same thing. You may have to go to somebody who is close to you and talk about this stuff. Maybe it's your parents, your spouse, your co-workers or a close friend. It may be time to sit down and talk about how you are changing for the better and how your relationship needs to change as well. But how do you do this the right way?

The first thing you have to do is confront the person. You have to be willing to say, "Listen, I value our relationship, but I can't live this way anymore. I have to start doing things differently. I want you to be on my team, but things have to change."

In Matthew 18:15, Jesus says, "If your brother sins against you, go and tell him his fault between you and him alone. If he hears you, you have gained your brother." You need to privately go to the person you need to confront and explain how you feel about him or her and how you feel about his or her influence in your life. Pray that God will open that person's eyes and ears to hear you, and that he or she will listen and desire to change with you. If the person does, you have gained a friend—a brother—who will be a valuable member of your team. I did this with my mother, and because she heard what I had to say, she is now one of my biggest supporters and encouragers.

The next thing you have to do is avoid or separate yourself from the people who are negatively impacting you. Psalm 1:1 offers this good advice: "Blessed is the man who walks not in the counsel of the ungodly, nor stands in the path of sinners, nor sits in the seat of the scornful." I had to learn to avoid those people who were trying to keep me from honoring God with my life and body. I had to avoid those people who were influencing me to eat more and to exercise less.

Now, some of you will argue that you can't avoid these people, because you live with them or work with them. This is true—you may not be able to avoid them completely or control their behavior. But you can control *yours*. This is where discipline kicks in: you have to learn to stop participating in destructive behavior. You must set the example of how to eat right, exercise more and live right. Just do your part, and then start praying that

God, your Coach, will convict these people to make the same positive changes in their lives. Lead by example, and let God do the rest.

Now, maybe you are saying to yourself, *I don't have to worry about this one. The people around me don't influence me that much. Their peer pressure doesn't affect me.* Well, I have news for you: that's just not true. The people with whom you surround yourself *do* impact you, for good or for bad. Let's talk about this a little bit, and then we'll see if you still feel the same way.

Friends Can Make You Fat!

One of the big health news stories in recent years was a study showing that a person's friends can influence the size of his or her waist (and the rest of that person's body). The study, coauthored by researchers from Harvard Medical School and the University of California at San Diego, revealed that a person's chances of becoming obese increase by 57 percent if a friend becomes obese, by 40 percent if a sibling became obese, and by 37 percent if a spouse became obese.[1] But why does this happen?

The major cause appears to be peer pressure. If your overweight friends think fat is beautiful, you may begin to think the same thing in order not to be left out. On the other hand, if thin is in with your friends, you may likely adapt to that attitude. From there, it's a short step to choosing food and exercise habits that will enable you soon look like the rest of the crowd—whether that means eating more food to look like your plus-sized friends or less food to look like your thin ones.

We need to find people with a common purpose and bond with those individuals in a commitment to shed pounds and get active. That's why team competitions are so valuable. Those folks on your team become your friends—your close friends who share your innermost thoughts. They are the ones who will hold you accountable in the tough times. They will be the first to slap you on the back when you are successful (even when it is only a tiny bit of success), and they will be the first ones to slap you in the face when you need a good wake up call to get back on track. When you make good choices, you not only help your waistline but also help your teammates, friends and family as well.

Another recent study published in the journal *Obesity* shows that overweight people, when compared to people of normal weight, are more likely to have overweight romantic partners (25 percent vs. 14 percent) and overweight best friends (24 percent vs. 14 percent). However, as researcher Tricia M. Leahey notes, "If your friends *expect* that you will eat healthy and exercise, this social pressure will likely lead you to eat healthy foods and engage in physical activity. . . . Having more people in your social network trying to lose weight [is] associated with increased motivation for weight loss."[2]

It doesn't take a rocket scientist to figure out what you need to do if you are trying to lose weight: surround yourself with people who want to eat healthy and exercise on a regular basis.

Watch Out! Colleagues Can Make You Fat!

As I've mentioned previously, co-workers can seriously sabotage your weight-loss efforts. There are retirement parties, birthday parties, company promotions (which always seem to involve food)—the list goes on and on. Add to that the huge boxes of sweets that vendors send during the holiday season in the hopes of securing your company's business for another year. Millions of calories later, your find yourself sorry you overindulged.

So, why did you eat all those calories when your every intent was to stay on track? It could be that your worst enemy wasn't in your pantry at home but sitting right next to you at work. After all, when a colleague brought in those homemade cookies to honor a teammate, you didn't want to appear non-supportive of the honoree. So you ate the treat, and then you paid for it in weight gain.

While teams of competitors can be tremendously helpful in losing weight, the opposite can also be true. Colleagues who don't want to face the fact you are being successful can sabotage your weight-loss efforts. Some of them might do this by predicting your imminent failure. "You'll probably just gain it all back," they say. "After all, my aunt did." Perhaps they do this because they are jealous, or they feel you have abandoned them at the table, or they just aren't disciplined enough themselves to refuse to eat the cupcake, donuts or apple strudel. They might even see the slimmer you as a threat to their job at the company.

Check Up

Big Belly = Less Money
An inverse relation between weight and socioeconomic status exists in affluent Western societies. Several studies have shown that obese or overweight workers in such nations are paid 1.4 to 4.5 percent less for the same job and work than their thinner counterparts. Furthermore, obesity and being overweight have been shown to have a potentially harmful effect on employment opportunities, income levels and social and public relationships.[3]

What's even harder than resisting a colleague is to say no to a client. Business lunches with a client can get pretty ugly when it comes to eating lightly. In fact, in a study conducted by the Medi-Weightloss Clinic, 1 in 5 participants said business lunches are where they feel the most pressure to overeat.[4]

You can't tell me that your friends, your co-workers and even your business client have no influence over you, because they do. We all want the affirmation and acceptance of those around us, and we tend to shy away from rocking the boat in those areas. But you have to learn how to negotiate the negativity in your life. You have to conduct those difficult conversations in your workplace and help people understand your new plan for living a healthier and better life. You have to come up with a line that pushes back at the food pushers, such as this one that Becky Hand, a registered dietitian with the weight-loss and fitness website SparkPeople, coaches people to say: "I've had your food in the past and it's always delicious. I'm sorry, but at this time in my life, eating those extra whatever isn't benefiting my health."[5]

When you avoid the unhealthy choices you see your co-workers making and refuse to submit to their negative peer pressure, you will lead by example and be a role model for them to follow. Once again, this won't be easy—but it will be necessary. So pray and ask God that your friends, family and colleagues at work will see your wiser and better choices and be motivated to make changes in their own lives.

Building Your Team

Once you have asked God to be on your team and dealt with the negative people in your life, you have to start surrounding yourself with positive people who are going to help you win. As motivational speaker James Rohn once said, "You are the average of the five people you spend the most time with." You are, in essence, who you hang out with, so you had better start looking at who these people are.

Proverbs 13:20 states, "He who walks with wise men will be wise, but the companion of fools will be destroyed. " If you walk with wise people, you will be wise; but if hang out with foolish people, you are going down. That's my take on it. It's time to decide with whom you are going to walk through life, and I challenge you to choose wise people for your team.

I really took this verse in Proverbs to heart, and I became determined to start looking for some wise people to start walking alongside me. After thinking a lot about how to go about doing this, I identified three areas where I needed help:

1. I needed to be *educated* in health and wellness and in eating and exercise.
2. I needed to be *encouraged* to make better choices.
3. I needed to be *equipped* for the journey.

I needed to identify people who could join my team and could help me in all areas of my life—spiritually, physically, socially and mentally. After all, I desired to be balanced and healthy in all of these areas. So I started looking at drafting people who would educate me, encourage me and equip me to be spiritually, physically, socially and mentally healthy.

Your Spiritual Team

While God needs to be number one in your life and your first draft pick, you also need to draft other people to help you stay on track spiritually. Talk with your pastor about your new outlook on life. Ask him to pray for you as you start to make these difficult changes. Also ask him to encourage you and to hold you accountable for how you take care of your body, the Temple of the Holy Spirit. Go to your small-group leader or Sunday School teacher and ask him to come alongside you and join your circle of support, praying for you and edifying you not to give up. This is what those in the Body of Christ are supposed to do for one another, but you have to be transparent and ask for their help and support. As I've mentioned before, it is so important to attend church and worship with other believers so you can be rejuvenated, recharged and persevere.

Your Physical Team

After God, your pastor and your church friends, your doctor needs to be your next draft pick. I can't drill home enough the importance of knowing where you are physically and what is your current state of health. This is a tough one for us guys, as we are notorious for not wanting to go to the doctor, but you have to get it into your head that your doctor must play an integral role on your team.

Men and Doctors

Because I am so passionate about this issue, I've put a lot of time and effort into studying the relationship between men and doctors. What I've found is that when it comes to men and health, they are their own worst enemies. "Many men are unaware that simple screening tests and lifestyle changes can dramatically improve their quality of life," says Dr.

Rick Kellerman, president of the American Academy of Family Physicians.[6] Thinking you are doing just fine and that nothing could ever happen to you is a symptom of classic denial. "A lot of times, it's very difficult for [men] to be convinced that they need to see a physician for a problem," says Dr. Allen Dollar, a cardiologist with Emory School of Medicine in Atlanta. "To a large extent, there is a lot of denial going on, and in some cases, that denial can be deadly."[7]

Some men don't want to face the possibility there could be something wrong with them. However, denial doesn't change the facts. You can deny there is a problem with your heart and then drop dead of a heart attack because you didn't go through some routine checkups. On the other hand, just because a family member died of heart failure, lung cancer or a brain tumor doesn't mean you will suffer from the same illness. So don't be afraid to go to the doctor and get something checked out. Even if there is a problem, it is surely better to be in contact with a doctor who can monitor you and help you deal with any eventuality.

Most health problems don't show up overnight. There are usually warning signs. Of course, if you are not doing routine care and are not aware of the symptoms of a disease, you are playing a dangerous game. Dr. David Dodson, an expert on men's health, recommends that healthy men under 50 get a regular checkup every 18 months. After 50, he suggests, men should see their doctors annually. "Men should take their health seriously," he says. "It's not just for their own sake. It's because men are part of families, and families depend on them."[8]

Many of the men interviewed in this book did not pay attention to their health until something traumatic happened in their lives that forced them to see their mortality. Again, I was one of them. I like how one writer puts it: "Due to macho pride or the expense of health care, many men visit the doctor only when something noticeably breaks, like their nose, or stops, like their heart."[9] In fact, experts believe the failure of men and doctors to meet on a regular basis could be one reason why women live longer than men and why men are more likely to die of serious diseases.

A Plan for Getting Started
If you are one of the guilty ones who almost never sees a doctor, here's a plan for getting started.

- *Stop the denial.* As I stated above, it is critical to not allow denial to keep you from getting regular checkups. "Men give lots of reasons why they avoid doctors, but some of the reasons they don't give are deeply embedded socially and culturally," explains Katherine Krefft, a psychologist who has dealt with this issue for years in her practice. "Many men have the attitude that what they don't know can't hurt them. That is rarely true about anything, but it can be especially dangerous when it comes to men's health."[10]

- *Get a doctor you can trust.* Find out who are the providers on your health plan. Insurance companies provide that information annually in booklet form or online, so find that information and start looking through it. Talk to friends who are satisfied with their physicians and ask them what they like about their doctors.

- *Determine you will get a checkup soon.* Some men find it easier to remember their annual physical exam if it is near another annual event, such as a birthday or an anniversary.

- *Recognize you are worth the time and money it takes to see a doctor.* Your family and friends need you and want you to stick around. So if you won't do it for yourself, at least do it for them.

- *Pick up the phone and make the appointment.* If you just cannot do it, get a family member to make the appointment for you—and then follow the instructions the doctor gives you!

- *Recognize that you are endangering your health if you do not see a doctor regularly.* The thinking that illnesses and problems will get better with time or with home remedies may not work if your body is harboring some serious condition.

Real men can and should go to the doctor. It's good for your health, and it's time to start setting a better example for the younger men in your life. Resolve to pick up the phone today and make that appointment.

Other Team Members
Other people you might want to consider adding to your team in the area of your physical health are nutritionists, physical therapists and personal trainers. These individuals all have valuable information to give you and can be valuable teammates. In appendix C in this book, I have dedicated a whole section to how to find a personal trainer. Also, make sure you read and reread the "Man Up" sections of this book, as they provide great tips from fitness and medical professionals that will help you get into shape.

Start praying that God will lead you to people who are going to help you improve your physical health.

Your Social Team

Your social network of support is important—don't forget what we talked about regarding how the people around you affect you. Start praying and asking God to send you people who will assist you in living a healthy life, and start looking for a network of people who are eating right and exercising. Put yourself out there on Facebook with your friends and with your family. Be open and transparent with people and tell them about your new goals. Ask them to hold you accountable to your plan.

I am sure you will be surprised at the amount of support and encouragement you receive. You might find some new friends who are struggling with the same things as you and who want to join you in this new game. You may become a role model to others who want to make the same changes. Sure, you might draw some criticism along the way, but we've already dealt with how to handle negativity. So start actively seeking a new network of support people who will push you to succeed.

Your Mental Team

Your mental team could consist of health care professionals and those who write about healthy living. While you may never meet these teammates, they still play an integral role in keeping you focused and on track. The cool thing about this team is that you can use technology and all kinds of different tools to keep you on track mentally.

Find your favorite periodical on healthy living and determine to read from it a few minutes each day. Listen to podcasts. Work out to music or download messages that will help keep your mind renewed, refreshed and inspired. Search for apps that can assist you. Listen to an audio version of the Bible while you exercise or just drive around in your car. Keep pouring positive things into your mind. You won't be sorry. The more you think on these things, the better chance you will have at success.

Join a Team of Losers

These are just a few examples of the types of people you can start drafting on your team to help you win. I'm sure you can think of a bunch of others to add to the list. One great place I suggest to help you find a lot of these people—and a great place to build an incredible circle of support—is a program called Losing to Live.

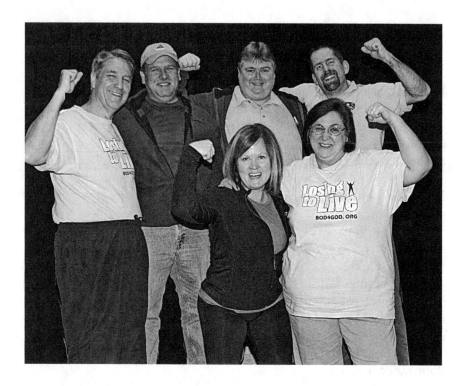

Losing to Live weight-loss competitions can be found in local churches all over the United States, and they are a great place to find people who share your goals in leading a healthy life. This faith-based weight-loss program was birthed out of my church, and currently we have collectively lost more than seven tons of weight. The program is based on a team approach to weight loss and healthy living.

As you read in several of the testimonials at the end of each chapter in this book, Losing to Live competitions take place over a 12-week time span, during which participants use my book *Bod4God: The Four Keys to Weight Loss*, the companion *Bod4God* DVD series, and group-starter tools to aid in meeting their weight-loss goals. Each participant is assigned to a team, which meets once a week. All the participants have the same goal: to fight obesity.

The competition offers participants an opportunity to lose weight in a fun and supportive environment. Each person is given two ways to approach the competition: personally or as a team. In the personal challenge, the person competes against himself or herself. In the team effort, the group members work together to encourage each other. There are three unique items about this program that make it so successful:

1. It is *biblical*: You learn how to apply the Bible to your weight-loss goals.
2. It is *personal*: You learn how to craft your own lifestyle plan.
3. It is *incremental*: You take small steps to life that slowly but surely lead you to a new place in weight and health.

In appendix D, I talk about Losing to Live in more detail and how you can find a Losing to Live competition to join or, if there isn't one in your area, how you can start one in your church. But don't just take my word for it. Listen to David Williams, one of my church's "losers" who has lost 92 pounds, tell you about how the Losing to Live program made a difference in his life and in the life of his family.

A little over a year ago, I weighed 344 pounds. I was dying—being crushed under my own weight. One night, I had a sleep apnea episode that frightened me. I remember that right before I fell asleep, I felt that I would not be coming back. I called out to the Lord to come get me, because I was sure I wouldn't wake up. Obviously, I did wake up, and the next morning I was soaked in sweat, extremely chilled and shaking all over. However, even with everything that had happened during that episode, I felt a peace that I had been saved. In that moment, I also knew I would have to do something to address my weight problem.

As it turns out, my wife and I were looking for a new church that had a great pastor of the Word. We were excited about Capital Baptist, and we joined the church. Later, we learned about the Losing to Live weight-loss competition that the church sponsored. I started the first level of the program in February 2011. It sounds funny, but even before I started the competition, I lost some weight. I like to think the Holy Spirit got me started. There is great peace and comfort in getting help from God and from a supportive church and program.

When you sign up for the Losing to Live weight-loss competition, you have a week to get ready. I love to read, so I went through *Bod4God*, which was part of the package along with a Losing to Live T-shirt. They took a photo of me in the shirt for the record, so that after I reached my weight goal they could take another shot for comparison.

I remember the first class held about a year ago. My leader was Rich Kay. Rich is in information technology, just as I am. He told me that because he had a real job, he couldn't go hopping over to the gym for a few hours whenever he felt like it. He also said he was

Before

After

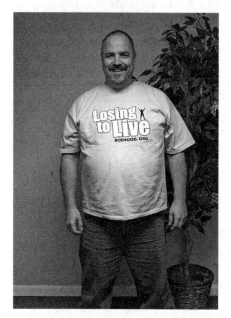
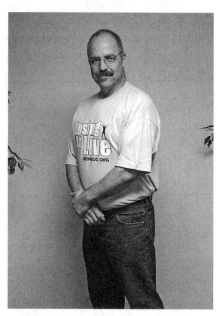

hooked on junk food, as many tech people are. Tech people have a lot of stress working with uncooperative computers and unhappy people, which can be very frustrating.

I had tried Nutri-System, Weight Watchers and other weight-loss programs in the past, and I had experienced some success with these, but I usually ended up gaining the weight back. This time, I was not fooled into thinking it would be an easy or quick fix. I hadn't accumulated the weight all at once, so I knew it would take time and patience to get it off. I was tired of suffering from severe sleep apnea and not being able to buy off-the-shelf jeans (unless the bigger sizes had just been restocked). I wanted to feel better about myself and be able to play sports again. So I decided, *I'm in!* I was excited and hopeful about the program, and I knew the support people around me would help me to be successful.

My biggest loss of 11.6 pounds in one week occurred during the second competition, and it happened because I was mindful of what I was putting in my mouth. Today I weigh 252 pounds, and my goal is 220.

I started excercising slowly and worked up. I now do ultimate cardio with Bob Harper's *Ultimate Strength*. It wasn't long before I was playing basketball and softball with the church teams. It was a wonderful moment when I hit my first softball and ran to first base. When I play basketball, we play 10 to 15-minute games, full court, and usually 4 to 5 games with about two- to four-minute breaks in between. Playing takes me back to some good high-school memories of competing in football and basketball. The other Saturday I nailed a sweet hook shot—nothing but net—and many of the men clapped and cheered. A banner moment in my quest for health occurred when my blood pressure dropped to 135/72 and my pulse was 58. I finally knew I was all right inside.

Each morning, I read a First Place 4 Health study and my Bible. The First Place 4 Health Bible Studies have recipes in the back, which is great because they helped me change the way I was eating. I'm not the cook in my home, so I went to my wife and asked her to cook healthier food, and she was willing to help me. The secret of getting her on board was to ask for her support and explain what I meant by cooking healthy. Now she and I not only eat together but also walk about three miles in the evenings. I have found that not only is it healthy to walk, but it is also a good time to work on issues relating to family and home.

Unlike other programs, Losing to Live includes God in the plan. This makes all the difference. If you are overweight, struggling and a Christian, ask God to help you. He will. He always does, and I thank Jesus Christ for all He has done in my life.

I truly hope my story helps you. I mean that. Always remember that you *can* change by making a strong commitment to yourself, joining a support group, and getting God's help.

Start Winning Together

I hope I have educated, encouraged and equipped you about the importance of drafting a team of people to help you achieve your goals. It is my prayer that I be counted among your list of teammates; someone who pushes you, just as Roy pushed me. That is the whole purpose of this book—to educate you on how to live a healthier life, encourage you along the way, and equip you with the tools necessary to complete the task. Let's start winning together. Let's make it a priority to get off the couch and get into shape. There is so much to be done in life and so many people to impact and influence. We must focus on the type of legacy we want to leave behind and for what types of things we want to be known. What do we want people to say about us when we've come to the end of our life?

How Are You Doing?

So, how are you doing? Are you tracking with the A.C.T.I.O.N steps? Are you *aware* of your physical condition? Ready to *commit* to change? Understanding that you have to *transform* your mind before you can transform your life? *Incorporating* small changes in your life to put you on the road to better health? How about joining an *organized* competition to help you *navigate* the journey to good health? That's what we're going to talk about next: how to navigate your way to good health.

Michael Parks
Drafts His Team

LOST 50 POUNDS

Before	After
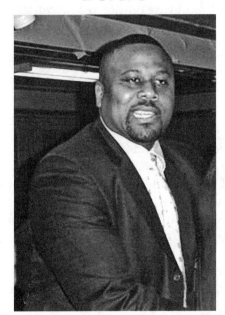	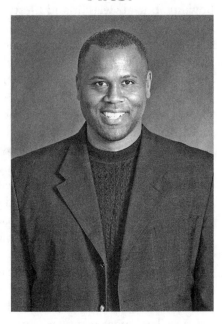

When I was growing up, we didn't have much, and that included food. I believe that because food was lacking, when I got to a place where I had food, I ate it until my weight ballooned.

I was small as a young person. In high school I was 4' 11" and weighed 89 pounds. I wanted to play football, but they wouldn't let me. I was just too small. So I started wrestling, and then I started to eat and eat. In high school, I went from 89 to 132 pounds. In college, I bulked up so I could wrestle in the 150-pound class in my junior year and the 158-pound class in my senior year. I kept gaining and gaining until I weighed 270 pounds.

Like Pastor Steve, I decided after college that if I never worked out again that would be fine, and I gained another 100 pounds. I knew I wasn't healthy, but the thought I might die didn't affect me. The prospect of death just wasn't enough to scare me into action. I reasoned that because I was a Christian, if I were absent from the body, I would be present with the Lord. I was being negligent with the body God had given me. What I was doing to my health was tantamount to putting a gun to my head.

I am an avid bowler, and at the time I was bowling a lot. I hurt my knee as a result of the repetitive bowling action, and I had a great deal of pain in that knee. I had an epiphany when I realized the problem was not the bowling, but my weight and lifestyle. I was living my life as a dehydrated man. I was dried up from the inside out.

I had been taking painkillers and all kinds of medicine, but I decided to stop taking everything and just live with the pain. But I hurt so much I could barely walk, let alone bowl. Finally, I started drinking water—lots of water. It was my first small step to life, and within two weeks the water accomplished what the medicine could not. I was pain free. Just by drinking water, I lost 20 pounds without exercising and without changing my diet.

Other than bowling, I didn't exercise until I found the Losing to Live weight-loss competition. At the time I worked at a school, and one of the organizers for activities approached me and said I would be perfect for karate. My knee was better, so I said yes, and I began taking karate lessons twice a week. It was amazing, because I did things I would never have been able to do before. I lost a few pounds, which was great, but I knew I also needed to get healthy.

Some time later, Pastor Steve came to our church for a men's conference. He gave me his phone number, and later on we connected and he asked if I would be interested in doing the Losing to Live weight-loss competition. I was not particularly interested at the time—I just wanted a copy of his book, *Bod4God: The Four Keys to Weight Loss*. Steve is all about progress, not perfection, and he asked my wife and me to come and talk with him. My wife got excited about everything he was doing, and she wanted to go through the whole program. So, that's what we did. By the time we finished, I had lost 26.2 pounds and my wife had lost 10.2 pounds.

Now we are second-generation losers. We launched a program in our own church last year, and our group lost a total of 300 pounds. We started our second program a few months later, and this second group has already exceeded the weight loss of the first group's total. I myself have lost a significant amount of weight, and I'm now at 220 pounds. My clothes are loose and I feel I look good, but I've become complacent. I've reached a plateau, and I know I have to do something about it because my goal is to get below 200 pounds.

I have a treadmill in my basement, but it's blocked by bowling balls and a lot of other stuff. I want to get to the treadmill . . . but I don't really want to get to it. I know that sounds like double talk and that if I *really* wanted to get to it, I'd move the stuff. The apostle Paul understood my dilemma. He said, "For what I am doing, I do not understand. For what I want to do, that I do not practice; but what I hate, that I do. . . . For the good that I will to do, I do not do; but the evil I will not to do, that I practice" (Romans 7:15,19). This weight-loss business is a spiritual journey.

In the past, I have treated my body like I treat my car. My car is not so clean. There are water bottles and papers on the seats and floor, which is okay with me, because it's my car. However, I can't treat my body in the same way, because it does not belong to me—it belongs to God. In the same way, the sooner you recognize that your body doesn't belong to you but to God, the sooner you will stop making excuses and get started on making it a healthy body for God's purposes.

Man Up

Eat Up: Plug in Positive Proteins

Replace heart-damaging red meat and pork with leaner poultry such as turkey or chicken. Better yet, eat Omega-3-rich fish, such as wild-caught salmon and sardines. Expand your horizons even more by trying some meals using plant proteins with beans, lentils or quinoa. Many studies show that high amounts of animal protein, including dairy, are linked to cancer growth, and cheese is full of salt and fat.[11] If you choose yogurt, get it plain without all the sugar and artificial flavors, and add your own fresh fruit.

Pump Up: Standard-Issue Push-ups

Push-ups set the standard for upper body strength training and use your own body weight. Lay face down with your hands shoulder-width apart and your chest and torso touching the floor. Put your legs together and put your weight on the balls of your feet. Push your entire body off the ground, completely locking your arms until there is no bend in your elbows, and then lower yourself to a starting position. Try it with your knees on the floor if this is too difficult to do. Do as many as you can, and then rest and repeat.

Reflection and Discussion Questions

1. In this chapter, we have examined how to make wise choices in drafting your teammates. Why is the wisest move making God your first draft pick?

2. In 1 Corinthians 15:33, Paul says, "Do not be deceived: 'Evil company corrupts good habits.'" In what ways do your friends and colleagues try to corrupt your good health habits?

3. It is important to draft a team of people who can help you in four critical areas of life: spiritually, physically, socially and mentally. In the space below, list people you can draft to help you in each of these areas.

   My spiritual team:

   My physical team:

My social team:

_____

_____

_____

_____

My mental team:

_____

_____

_____

_____

4. Who do you need to confront to get rid of negativity in your life? Who do you need to avoid?

_____

_____

_____

_____

5. When was your last doctor's visit? What did you learn, and how has it impacted you and your health?

_____

_____

_____

_____

_____

6. Proverbs 27:17 says that the people around you will sharpen you. Are your overall relationships having a positive or negative influence on your health?

_____

_____

_____

_____

MY PERSONAL GAME PLAN FOR

GETTING IN SHAPE

*Beloved, I pray that you may prosper in all things
and be in health, just as your soul prospers.*

3 JOHN 2

This book is about **ACTION** and about **DOING**! In the spaces below, record what actions you are going to take to improve your health this week.

Aware—I will do the following to show I am aware of my current physical condition and that my body matters to God:

_____
_____
_____
_____
_____

Commit—I will do the following to commit to living a disciplined life and to winning over temptation:

_____
_____
_____
_____
_____
_____

Transform—This is how I will transform the way I think and live:

_____
_____
_____
_____
_____

Incorporate—I will incorporate these healthy eating habits and exercise into my daily life:

_____

_____

_____

_____

_____

Organize—This is how I will organize a team of people to help me win:

_____

_____

_____

_____

_____

Navigate—This is my action plan for healthy living and navigating my way to leaving a lasting legacy:

_____

_____

_____

_____

_____

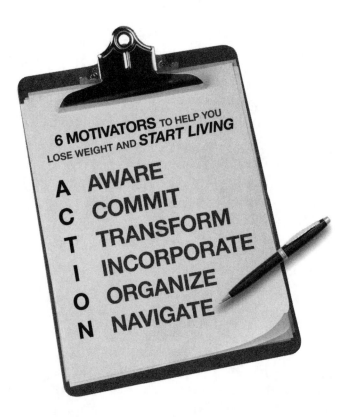

6 MOTIVATORS TO HELP YOU LOSE WEIGHT AND START LIVING

A AWARE
C COMMIT
T TRANSFORM
I INCORPORATE
O ORGANIZE
N NAVIGATE

Navigate

The fifth and final step in your journey is to create an A.C.T.I.O.N. plan for healthy living so you can *navigate* your way to leaving a lasting legacy. You only have one life—one that is too valuable to waste—so it's time to start putting a plan together that will help you live longer and continue to impact and influence the lives around you. It's important to finish well, so keep your eyes on the endzone and head for it, giving it everything you've got.

Chapter 11

Make Your Dash Count

I have fought the good fight, I have finished the race, I have kept the faith.
2 TIMOTHY 4:7

"Gramma, when I grow up, I'm gonna play football for the Green Bay Packers, just like Bart Starr. You wait and see!"

That was my boyhood dream. It was what I wanted more than anything . . . well, that and to become Superman. Actually, I didn't see any reason why I couldn't do both. I could be a football player by day and a superhero by night. Those were the dreams and fantasies I played out during the summers of my childhood, many of which were spent on my Gramma Emma's farm in southern Virginia.

Do you remember those lazy days of summer when the only worry or care you had was what new adventure would be found that day or how you could scrounge up enough money to buy ice cream, soda or baseball cards? Do you remember those days spent fishing, riding bikes, playing football and cops and robbers, and playing in the creek? Back then, what determined a truly great day was how dirty you were by the end of it or how exhausted you were when you finally collapsed into your bed at night. It was a time of adventure, fun and dreams—dreams of the future and what you wanted to be when you grew up.

What little boy doesn't dream of being a superhero, or a professional football player, or an astronaut, or a soldier? That overwhelming desire to have an impact and make a difference seems to carry with us into adulthood. It is as if God has wired men to conquer, be adventurous and take risks. We are still little boys at heart, looking for the chance to save the day.

Steve Reynolds

But as we grow up, boyhood dreams and fantasies fade away and become fond—but distant—memories of our past. As we mature and take on more responsibilities, we have less time to play and dream. Summer vacations that used to last three months turn into summer jobs, and then into just one or two weeks if we are lucky. However, just because we have less time to play doesn't mean we should stop dreaming of adventure and of being conquerors.

We don't have to be little boys to dream big dreams and have ambitious goals. True, we can't become superheroes in real life with superhuman strength and abilities, but who says we can't be a hero to those around us? Why can't we be someone who influences others to do good? Why can't we encourage others to achieve more? Wouldn't it be great to be a guy who helps those around him when they are in need and serve as a role model for others to follow? That's a real hero.

It's important to never stop dreaming. In fact, the older you get, the more you need to keep doing it. You need to remember what it felt like to be a little boy living in that world of fantasy so you can get in the right frame of mind to start dreaming again. You need to start thinking about what you want to accomplish in life and the people you can help along the way. So get out that pillowcase—you know, the one you tied around your neck as your superhero cape—and get ready to jump off your bed. Get ready to fly!

Ready for Adventure!

I couldn't wait for the last day of school to arrive. I wanted to be free from all the classes, homework, tests and schedules. I was ready for adventure to begin.

The approach of summer meant my parents would be taking me to the home of Emma Reynolds, my paternal grandmother. My grandfather, Homer Reynolds, had died when I was just a young boy. Gramma Reynolds needed help on the farm, so my cousin Dillard and I would go there during the summer break to help out. Yes, there was a lot of hard work involved, but there were also many fun and exciting things to do—things I couldn't do at home. Many of my fondest childhood memories revolve around those long summer visits.

Down behind my grandmother's house was a pond stocked with fish. Dillard and I, wearing our cut-off jeans and T-shirts, would grab a couple of bamboo sticks for poles. We would dig up some worms, throw them in a cup, and head to the pond to catch us some fish. We looked like a couple of little rascals—except I wasn't so little. We usually caught something. When we did, we would run back to the house with our fish so Gramma could fry them up and feed them to us, along with eggs and toast. It was delicious. We were two proud young fishermen enjoying our catch of the day.

Dillard and I also loved to pretend we were superheroes like Batman, Robin and Superman. Now, don't judge me. I know you secretly wanted to be like a superhero too. Maybe you wanted to be Spiderman or Captain America. In any event, we would run all over that farm, pretending to rid the world of injustice by fighting for good against the evil villains. We also played a lot of football in the front yard. On Sunday afternoons, my Uncle Ralph would come over and throw the football to us for what seemed like hours. I became a football player at an early age, and those dreams I had of making it big and playing in the NFL were vivid and real to me.

However, as I said, even though Dillard and I were on summer vacation, our days weren't all filled with fun and games. It was a working farm, which meant we had a lot of work to do during the day. Our list of chores was long and included everything from baling hay, cutting and hauling wood, cleaning, weeding, picking food from the garden, digging potatoes, gathering corn and strawberries, harvesting tobacco, feeding the cows and canning and preserving food. It was hard work, and I remember falling into bed at night exhausted. I would pull up the most comfortable quilts imaginable—ones that Gramma had made—and I'd be asleep in seconds. The feeling of satisfaction, of a job well done, and the sense of home was incredible.

Boyhood Lessons

I learned some valuable lessons during those summers that I carried with me into adulthood. First and foremost, I learned to love nature and the beauty of God's creation. The world was my playground, and it seemed as if God had created it just for me. I savored and enjoyed every bit of it. I learned the value and necessity of farming and just how hard farmers work. I learned to appreciate the way we get our food. It's amazing to plant a seed and watch in wonder as it grows to maturity and is ready to harvest. It is so satisfying to walk out to the garden and pick food that you planted yourself and eat it. To this day, I love farm-fresh produce and vegetables, and every time I eat a tomato right from the garden, it takes me back to my summers on the farm.

I also learned to work hard. There wasn't any slacking allowed at Gramma's house. You had to do your share, and Dillard and I knew we wouldn't be allowed to play until all of our chores were done. In fact, both my Gramma Reynolds and my parents instilled in me the value of hard work at an early age. I remember one time when my father and I were cutting pulp wood to sell. We had to cut each tree into five-foot sections. It was hard, physical labor, and those sections were heavy and difficult to lift. At one point, I looked up at my father and said, "Daddy, I don't know what I'm gonna be when I grow up, but I do know this: I'm not gonna cut wood!" Nobody worked harder than my parents and my grandparents to give their family the best, and while I stuck to my promise of not cutting wood when I grew up, I did adopt the work ethic they passed on to me.

During those summers, my love and appreciation for my family was strengthened. I was able to spend quality time with my parents, my grandmother and my extended family and build memories that will last a lifetime. I will never forget Sunday afternoons after church when everyone would come to Gramma's house for lunch. It seemed she cooked for an army that day—it wasn't unusual for her to feed up to 25 people. She spent hours making incredible food like fried chicken, ham, potatoes and gravy, fish, green beans, corn pudding, potato salad, squash, fresh tomatoes, fried green tomatoes, German chocolate cake, and berry and custard pies.

Sunday dinner looked like a huge banquet, and to me it felt like heaven. We also made homemade ice cream, taking turns cranking the old-fashioned ice cream maker. I think this is where my love for ice cream was born. My family would sit around that table, talking, laughing, eating and having a great time just enjoying being with one another. After dinner we would play cards and board games, throw the football around, and play crochet on the front lawn. We enjoyed being with one another and just living life.

Yet the most important lesson I learned during those times spent at Gramma's house was to love God. After a long, hard day of work and adventure, Dillard and I would sit in Gramma's humble living room and listen while she read from the Bible. She would sit there in her old flannel nightgown with all this goop on her face. She smelled to high heaven, and she looked kind of like the villains we superheroes had been fighting that day. Her voice was as sweet as it could be as she poured into us the truth from God's Word.

As I look back on those moments, I realize that the time Gramma spent with me was an investment in my life that has paid huge dividends. Not only did she read the Bible to Dillard and me, but she also made sure we were in church every Sunday—and that we attended Vacation Bible School as well. It was important to her (and to our family) that we were brought up in church and that we learned to love God.

I gave my heart to God in Gramma's little country church, New Hope Baptist, and my life was never the same from that point on. My parents helped cultivate the seeds of truth planted at this early stage of my life, and they continued to invest in my spiritual life by helping me grow in my relationship with God. They took me to church and made sure I lived a godly life. Later on, they sent me to a Christian university. In fact, I don't know where I would be today if they hadn't been committed to helping me become a godly man.

A Man in the Making

Those times at the farm and the lessons my family taught me have helped mold me into the man I am today. The legacy of faith and family that was passed down to me by my parents and grandparents has stuck with me all these years, and it is a legacy that I am working to pass on to my kids and my future grandkids. My walk with Christ began during those early years, and it has continually grown since then. It led me to dedicate my life to serving God as a pastor, giving of myself daily to influence others, lead people to Christ, and touch the lives of individuals all over the world.

I don't know what was going through my Gramma Emma's mind as she was reading to Dillard and me. I don't think she had any idea that I would one day pastor a large church right outside Washington, DC. I doubt she ever fathomed that I would appear on TV, radio and in newspapers to talk about my weight-loss journey, or even that one day I would be writing a book mentioning the influence she had on me. She was a simple woman who lived a simple life, and she loved her grandsons and just wanted them to know about the God she loved.

It's easy to see the influence that Gramma Reynolds had on our family. She first passed her faith on to my father, Alfred, and then to my mother, Betsy, who then passed it on to me and my brother, Donald. Grandma Reynolds was a hero in my life, and I am deeply committed to being a hero in the same way to my children, Crystal, Sarah and Jeremiah. I want to pass on to my children and future generations the legacy I received from my family. I want them to love God and love their family more than anything. To do this, I know I have to lead a healthy life so I can be around to teach them the important lessons my parents and grandparents taught me. I want to be an active part of their lives.

During those summers on the farm, Gramma was right there doing chores with us and working as hard as we were. She was engaged in our lives, and this is how I want to live my life. I want to work hard and love

235

Steve Reynolds

hard until my last breath. I want to finish well. But how does one do this? How does a person finish his or her life well?

It's About Finishing Well

Leaving a legacy doesn't happen by accident—there are certain things you must do to finish well. As Ecclesiastes 3:2 tells us, there is "a time to be born, and a time to die," which means we cannot escape the fact that just as we were born, one day we are going to die. The only thing we have control over is what we do with our life in the meantime.

There is an old saying that when you look at a tombstone, there are two dates inscribed on it: the birth date of the person buried there and the date that person died. But in the middle of those two dates is a little dash, which signifies all the years that passed between those two dates. That dash stands for everything that is crucial to you finishing well. It stands for everything you did with your life. So, I ask you, when you come to the end of your life, what do you want your dash to say about you?

I love the way the apostle Paul—a superhero of the Bible—talks about the end of his life in 2 Timothy 4:6-7: "For I am already being poured out as a drink offering, and the time of my departure is at hand. I have fought the good fight, I have finished the race, I have kept the faith." Wow! Those were likely his final words just before he was beheaded and martyred for Jesus.

What was Paul feeling? What was he thinking about? He was thinking about finishing well. He told Timothy that he had fought hard for the

Check Up

Big Belly = Low Life

It is a fact that a person's quality of life suffers when he or she is obese or overweight. Obese adults have more annual admissions to the hospital, more outpatient physician visits, higher prescription drug costs, and worse health-related quality of life than individuals with normal weight. Certain medical conditions such as obstructive sleep apnea, back pain, joint pain, diabetes and hypertension are clearly related to elevated body mass indices. Obese individuals are also more easily fatigued. Not only are these conditions more prevalent in obese and overweight individuals, but also they are often more serious and difficult to manage medically, requiring more medications and more interventions. In addition, heart disease in obese individuals carries a higher mortality rate. A study conducted in 2002 indicates that the health risks of obesity are greater than smoking or heavy drinking.[1]

cause of Christ and that he had finished what God wanted him to do—and that he continued to believe in Jesus the entire time he was doing it. That's what I want people to say about me after I'm gone. I desire to have that same testimony, and I hope you do as well.

But in order to end well, you need to ask yourself these questions: *What kind of departure will I have? Will I leave this life because of disease? Will I develop health and physical conditions that will kill me? Will I die of something I could have prevented if I had just taken better care of my body? Or will I lead a life that allows me to be an influence on my family for years to come?* These are powerful questions you need to start considering, because you can't focus on how you are going to finish well until you have honestly answered them. In the next few pages, I will share my strategy for finishing well.

Seek a Long Life

The first thing you need to do is to seek a long life. Yes, that's right: you have to *want* to live a long time. Here's how I look at this. When it comes to finishing well, I believe duration—simply surviving—matters. While history tells us of people who weren't on this earth for very long and yet made a huge impact with their lives, I believe the longer a person is in this world, the greater difference he or she can make. The longer a person is around, the more people he or she can invest in with a greater impact. So, I have decided to seek a long life.

My prayer is that I will live to be at least 100 years old. I actually pray that God will allow me to live that long! The good news is that current trends are on my side. In fact, the last census shows that the number of people who live to be at least 100 years is rising, and that by the year 2050, there will be approximately 601,000 people who are at least 100![2] I want to be a part of that crowd. I want the duration of my life to be as long as possible so I can do more with it. I want to tell more people about Jesus, train more people to do God's work, and help as many people as possible achieve a healthier and more productive lifestyle. But, most important, I want to invest in my family so future generations of Reynolds can impact and change lives as well. Are you praying that God will give you a long life so you can do the same?

Along with my prayer to live to be 100, I also have a plan for how to do it. That plan has a lot to do with my lifestyle. Now, I know what you are saying right now: "God is in control of when we die!" You are right. However, we have a lot of control over the way in which we live and whether or not we choose to kill ourselves with our poor choices and bad habits.

When I weighed 340 pounds, I brought disease upon my body. I had high blood pressure (the silent killer), high cholesterol (which clogged my arteries) and diabetes (which threatened my life). I had to wake up and face the fact that I was going to die—and soon—if I didn't change my ways.

My problem was that I had a bod for Steve. However, once I went to the Bible to see what I needed to do to get healthy again, I realized I needed to change my plan to having a bod for God. I had to surrender my fork to God, start eating less, and start exercising more. As I relate in my book *Bod4God,* when I did, the problems with my high blood pressure and high cholesterol levels went away, and *I no longer suffered from type-2 diabetes.*

Make a Significant Impact

In order to finish well, you need to make a significant impact on others. Like the apostle Paul, you need to fight "the good fight" (2 Timothy 4:7). But what did Paul mean by this? Well, he was talking about life. Life is often difficult. There will be suffering, hardship, pain and betrayal. As Paul states in Acts 14:22, "We must through many tribulations enter the kingdom of God." The Christian life is not going to be easy, but you must fight, endure and persevere. You can't quit.

Don't give in to Satan. Don't give up. Don't throw in the towel and become known as someone who gave up and never succeeded in reaching his goals. Be remembered as a fighter who gave this life all he had and went down swinging. Getting off that couch and getting back into the game of life will not be easy, but you must do it. You must be determined to honor God with your life and your body and commit yourself to doing His will, not yours. You will never be sorry that you stayed in the fight, but if you quit, you will regret it forever.

Making a significant impact means finishing the race—the course—and not giving up halfway. This requires direction. First, you have to live your life *under* the direction of God, and then *in* the direction He wants you to go with your life. In Acts 20:24, Paul says, "But none of these things move me; nor do I count my life dear to myself, so that I may finish my race with joy." Paul didn't just want to just finish the race; he wanted to finish it with *joy.* He wanted to finish what God had given him to do. In the same way, you want to go to the grave knowing you accomplished everything God had for you—whatever that might look like in your life—for this leads to true joy. You might not do everything on your list, but make sure you accomplish everything God wants you to do. That is finishing well!

Finally, guys, you need keep the faith. A significant life has everything to do with your relationship with God, and the only way you are going to be able to fight the good fight is if you are rooted and grounded in the truth of God's Word and growing in your relationship with Him. It is also the only way you are going to know what God wants you to do with your life. Remember that you were made by God and for God. Your body was created to glorify Him and do His service. Without faith, nothing you do in this life matters. As the writer of Hebrews 11:6 says, "But without faith it is impossible to please Him." You have to forge faith and fitness together so you can have strength for the journey and accomplish all God has for you to do.

Coming Full Circle

This past Thanksgiving, my family and I went back to Gramma Reynolds's farm. Things had changed over the years since Gramma passed away. The house and buildings were showing their age, the fields were overgrown, and everything seemed much smaller to me now that I was grown. It was different than the way I remembered it, and yet it all seemed so familiar. But the feelings and emotions the place brought out in me were still the same, and I found myself getting choked up.

My parents were there with Debbie and me, and so were my three children and my son-in-law. I spent quite a bit of time walking around, reminiscing with them about those long-lost days of summer—the summers of my youth. I could see myself in so many different places around the farm: playing in the yard and at the pond, working in the fields, sitting on the front porch with Gramma.

After we spent some time exploring, we decided to head over to the gravesite of my grandparents, Homer and Emma. There, my son, Jeremiah, and I and my father stood together at the gravesite of my grandfather, Homer—four generations of Reynolds men. It was an incredible moment

in my life, and one that I will never forget. Even though I never knew Homer, according to my father he was a godly man. He was a man who taught his eight children the same lessons my parents taught me: to work hard, appreciate your family, and love God. He was a loving, kind and patient man who always had

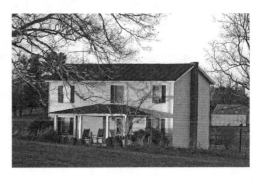

something encouraging and positive to say. He was an incredible father and husband and was dedicated to his family, his farm and his church.

Even though my grandfather wasn't able to have a physical presence in my life, his legacy of faith and family were passed on to me, and, as I have said, I am striving to pass them along to my children. Whereas in the days of my youth my superheroes were Batman, Robin and Superman, now my superheroes are my parents and grandparents. If I am able to be half the parent to my children that they were to me, I will be successful in my eyes. I want to continue what they started so many years ago, and I want to see the legacy continue to be passed from generation to generation.

Standing there that day at the gravesite made me really think about my "dash" and what I want people to say about me at my grave. Did I finish well? Did I live a life of significance? Did it all matter? I want to make my dash count. I want to be on earth as long as I can and influence my family until my dying breath. In the same way, I want to challenge you to do whatever it takes to leave a legacy. Be a hero. Hey, you can even wear a cape if you want to do so! Put on those "super dad," "super husband" and "super friend" T-shirts and start fighting for good against the forces of darkness. Just do me one favor: please don't put on tights!

Get the Game Plan

We've nearly come to the end of our time together, but before I leave you, I want to give you a game plan for health—a road map for *navigating* the rest of your life. So stay with me to the last page of the book. There is much more practical help here for you!

Pastor Jim Goforth
Dreams for a Healthier Future

LOST 54 POUNDS

Before	After

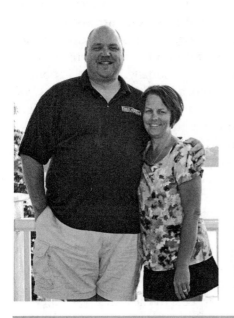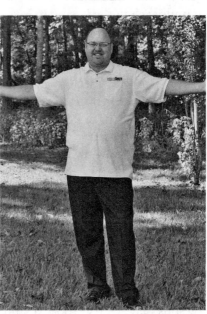

When I became a Christian, I was in great shape physically, even though before my conversion all I did was drink beer and smoke pot. When I stopped all that stuff, I started gaining weight. The problem grew worse when I became a pastor, because in our circles it is all right to go out after every service and eat and eat. I was an emotional eater, and I would go without food all day long and then eat enough at night to equal a full day of meals. I ate to relieve stress and to calm my nerves.

It took a series of events in my life to finally get my attention and make me want to change. One was that I went to the doctor and was diagnosed with high blood pressure and diabetes. In fact, the doctor called me "morbidly obese." That was hard to hear, and I didn't respond well. I got ticked off rather than motivated. The doctor wanted me to go on medication, but

I refused. He said, "I'll give you six months to change and then put you on medication." I was afraid, and for the first time in my life I felt fragile. I have two great kids and I wanted to be around for them, but I didn't know how to change. After five months had passed and I still hadn't done anything about my weight, I was feeling the crunch of the six-month deadline.

Then I met Pastor Steve at an advanced coaching network for pastors. When he told me about his weight-loss journey, something clicked. There were three or four other pastors at the conference who had lost about 80 pounds each in the Losing to Live competition. That got my attention, so I decided to give the program a try and make the commitment to do the program at our church. Two hundred and five people signed up, and Pastor Steve came and introduced the competition to our congregation. It was life-changing for our people and for me personally. I've lost 54 pounds so far, and our groups have lost a combined weight of more than 1,000 pounds. There have been other side benefits in addition to the weight loss—my congregation thinks I'm more energized. Maybe I am. I just know the church is growing again. Something has changed.

The Losing to Live plan works where other diet plans fail because it establishes a connection between the head and the heart. The truth is that we're made by God and for God is a strong motivator. I learned quickly that by not taking care of my body, not only was I destroying myself, but I was also offending my Creator.

My wife and sons have been supportive of my involvement with the Losing to Live competition. My wife had already lost some weight, and my getting on the weight-loss program only motivated her to do more. One of my sons plays college football and the other is in the military, so they are both into health and fitness. Now my wife and I are getting into shape as well, and we're about to run our first 5K race.

Today, we're serious at our church about getting people healthy. We've put in a track where people can walk or run. It's inspiring to see the folks out there. And not only do they walk for health, but they also establish new relationships as they are walking. People from outside the church also come to the track, and to date six people have come to Christ through our efforts to get a healthy congregation. We let those who do not regularly attend our church know about the upcoming competitions through direct mail. We send a piece to everyone in the community.

I would like to encourage you to get on the road to help by doing *something*, no matter how small that action might be. In our church we have a saying that "every step toward God is a good one." My first small step was to cut my meals in half. When I ate out, before I ever started to eat anything

I asked for a container and divided the food into two portions. It worked for me, and it's exciting to find a new way to live.

We had such a huge and unanticipated response to our first competition that we needed more groups and more leaders. People I would have never expected to show interest in leadership stepped up to lead. Amazing! The competition helped my church understand that there are other ways to meet the needs of people in our community than just preaching. There were ways we had never dreamed about.

I have a great passion to see my congregation healthy and strong. We are thinking about some new ways of helping people outside our church circle get healthy, and find Christ. I would like to see more play structures for the kids in town. I would like to have some exercise equipment for the Losing to Live competitors and maybe see corporate people come in for events and use the equipment. Because health is such huge problem in this country, we in the Church—in the Body of Christ—have a huge opportunity to help others not only live long lives, but also live for all eternity.

Man Up

Eat Up: Ban MSG

Monosodium glutamate, or MSG, is your enemy! Research shows a strong connection between consuming MSG and developing obesity. And those who eat foods with this flavor enhancer end up not only consuming more calories by the end of the day but also damaging the neurons in their brain. I don't know about you, but I need all the brain cells I have! So read the ingredients list, and if MSG is there (it is present in almost all processed food), don't buy the product.

Pump Up: Jump-start Your Heart

Jumping jacks are total body exercises that rev up your heart rate while working your lower leg muscles and your abdominal muscles. Begin by standing with your arms at your side. Bend your knees and jump as you spread your feet shoulder-width apart and move your arms in a circular motion at the same time. Jump again and return to your starting position. If you physically cannot do a jumping jack, a low-impact alternative can be done while sitting on the edge of a chair. Keeping your knees and feet together, raise them about six inches off the floor, and then hold that position as you do the arm movements for a jumping jack. Do 10 repetitions, rest, and then do 10 more.

Reflection and Discussion Questions

1. Are you satisfied with your life as it is now—with the dash you are living? Why or why not?

2. Every guy loves the idea of making an impact. What are some of the ways you want to make an impact with your life?

3. If someone interviewed your child about what kind of parent you are and the kind of example you set, what would your child say?

4. Longevity doesn't just happen. What is your game plan for living a long life?

5. What type of legacy do you desire to leave for your family? How will you go about leaving this legacy behind for them?

_____

_____

_____

_____

_____

6. In 2 Timothy 4:7, Paul says we must fight the good fight, finish the race, and keep the faith. How does this relate to making your dash count?

_____

_____

_____

_____

_____

MY PERSONAL GAME PLAN FOR

GETTING IN SHAPE

*Beloved, I pray that you may prosper in all things
and be in health, just as your soul prospers.*

3 JOHN 2

This book is about **ACTION** and about **DOING**! In the spaces below, record what actions you are going to take to improve your health this week.

Aware—I will do the following to show I am aware of my current physical condition and that my body matters to God:

_____

_____

_____

_____

_____

Commit—I will do the following to commit to living a disciplined life and to winning over temptation:

_____

_____

_____

_____

_____

_____

Transform—This is how I will transform the way I think and live:

_____

_____

_____

_____

_____

Incorporate—I will incorporate these healthy eating habits and exercise into my daily life:

_____

_____

_____

_____

_____

Organize—This is how I will organize a team of people to help me win:

_____

_____

_____

_____

_____

Navigate—This is my action plan for healthy living and navigating my way to leaving a lasting legacy:

_____

_____

_____

_____

_____

Chapter 12

Your Game Plan for Health

Then the LORD *answered me and said: "Write the vision and make it plain on tablets, that he may run who reads it."*
HABAKKUK 2:2

I clearly remember walking into my locker room at Liberty University just before I played the last game of my college football career. It was an emotional moment. My team was energized. It was hard to believe that this was it . . . the last time we would take the field. We were fired up to win. We wanted victory so bad that we could taste it. Our focus was on ending the season strong, on a high note. We weren't going to let anything get in our way or hinder us from achieving our goal. There wasn't the usual joking or fooling around. This game was much too important for that, and we knew it.

An eerie silence settled on the room. You could hear the locker doors slamming and the sounds of the ripping tape as we geared up. We put on our game faces and began to prepare our minds for what we were about to do. We listened to our coach as he gave us the typical pre-game talk. It went kind of like this: "Guys, it's time to fight! This is what you have worked for. When you get out on that field, remember what you're supposed to do. They want to take you down. You can't let them get up on ya. Let them know who we are and what we are here to do. Own that field. Dominate it! Don't give them an inch."

The coach's talk was meant to pump us up and get us to take care of business out on the field. But he went on to say something different that day—something that has stuck with me all these years. He spoke directly to the seniors on the team and told us that this was our last game. He challenged us to make this one game count—it was one more chance to win. That was a powerful moment for me. I realized I might never again play this game that I loved so much; the game that had been such an integral part of my life. It made me want to give even more when I got out there on that field, and that thought made me push myself harder once I got in the game.

This same thought is what I want to leave you with as we close this book. You may have only one more shot at getting your physical condition under control—one more shot to change before something bad happens. You only have one life to live, so don't waste it. You have to play to win and make this game count. Your life depends on it. So, much like my coach at Liberty, I want to "write the vision and make it plain" for you (Habakkuk 2:2). I want to leave you with my locker-room pep talk to get you fired up and focused on what *you* need to do.

It's Your Turn

The great thing, guys, is that as you read my pep talk, you get to miss out on all the painful stuff that I had to endure during my pre-game locker room moments in college. You'll miss out on the physical torture I went through, such as slapping each other around, punching one another, banging our helmets together (after they were already on . . . that one wasn't very smart!). And don't forget the butt slapping. I'll just stick to the motivational and practical stuff (you can thank me later) and give you a strategy on how to stay focused on your goals—on how to *win*.

Play to Win

Pretend right now I'm screaming at you and saying, "PLAY TO WIN!" It's not enough to just start something; that's the easy part. If you are running a race, those first few minutes after the gun goes off are a piece of cake. It's the middle of the race—when the starting line is far from sight and the finish line seems so far away—that the physical and mental fatigue set in and the urge to quit takes root.

It's the same way with weight loss and getting in shape. Hopefully, at this stage of the game you are feeling pumped up and motivated to get off that couch and get moving. The hard part is being consistent, staying focused on your goals, and working to achieve them for the long run. You have to learn how to keep your focus on doing the right thing all the time.

In 1 Corinthians 9:24, Paul says, "Do you not know that those who run in a race all run, but one receives the prize? Run in such a way that you may obtain it." I love that last part: "Run in such a way that you may obtain it." Paul is stating that an athlete has to stay focused if he is going to win. The same thing applies to you when it comes to getting in shape. You need to have the mentality that you are in it to win it and that you are playing to win. If you have this mindset, you will be much more focused and have a much greater chance of achieving the goals you set for yourself.

Weight loss can be a rollercoaster with lots of ups and downs. Let's face it: all of us at one time or another have tried to lose weight only to gain it back (and then some). Why did we fail? Because we didn't stay focused on the goal—on winning. We waste so much time in our lives because we don't stay focused. The good news is that unlike in a footrace where there is only one winner, in this new game we are starting to play, *everyone* can win. We all can integrate new strategies and habits that will produce positive changes and result in us leading healthier lives. That's winning!

The Desire to Win

There are two keys to playing to win: passion and endzone thinking. First, you have to have a desire to win. You have to want it so badly that you are willing to do the hard work necessary for success. When you are exhausted on that treadmill and in pain from working out muscles you haven't used in a long time, passion will keep you going. When you are tempted to cheat and pull into a fast food drive-thru after a long day of work, passion will help you steer that car in the opposite direction. You can't win without passion, and you can't live without it. It is what's going to keep you moving in the right direction.

One of the characteristics of people who don't want to waste their lives is that they are so passionate about their goals that they are willing to eliminate whatever they must in order to win. Sometimes this involves making hard decisions in life, such as eliminating negative relationships that may be holding them back. At other times, it may mean taking a hard look at their lives and getting rid of things that are keeping them from changing. I hope that after reading this book, you are starting to feel this fire igniting inside of you—a passion for getting up and getting in shape.

Endzone Thinking

The second thing you have to do in order to play to win is begin with the end in mind. I call this endzone thinking. You have to picture yourself at the end of the game, holding the trophy and celebrating your victory. You have to focus on doing that endzone dance and spiking the football.

251

People who train for marathons use this strategy when preparing for the race. They study the route of the course, analyze where their pit stops will be, and identify hills and other obstacles they will have to overcome. They visualize themselves crossing the finish line again and again. They focus on the end and winning the race. You need to do the same.

Begin by focusing on the end result of reaching your goals. What are you going to look like at that point? What are you going to feel like? You are going to look better, feel better and generally be healthier, so picture that in your mind. Envision having a better quality of life and being able to do more. Keep these images in your mind during the tough times and write down all the things you are going to do to celebrate once you get there. Keep your eyes and mind fixed on the prize.

Next, focus on the end of your life, when you will stand before Jesus and give an account of what you have done during your time on earth. In 2 Corinthians 5:10, Paul says, "For we must all appear before the judgment seat of Christ, that each one may receive the things done in the body, according to what he has done, whether good or bad." This is a sobering thought—you are going to have to give an account for what you did with your body. I know that once the full implication of this verse set in with me, I started focusing on taking better care of myself!

I want to be able to stand before Jesus and say I did my best to take care of the body He gave me—the one I used to do His work on earth. I want to know that I maximized it and didn't waste it, trash it or pollute it with the things I put in it. I want you to be able to do the same thing. So focus not only on the time when you have achieved your goals but also on that day when you will be standing before Jesus to give an account for how you lived. Play to win.

Pay the Price

You don't become a successful quarterback in the NFL without dedicating your life to being a champion. For a football player, it isn't just something you do in the fall. You don't play with a little ball for two or three months and then quit. No, football controls your life every day, year round, day in and day out. The rigors of being an athlete—the diet and exercise regimen you have to maintain—costs something. You pay the price if you choose this type of lifestyle.

College football players have the added burden of having to maintain good grades. When I played at Liberty, the school was heavily committed to having its athletes maintain good academics, because the school knew most of us wouldn't make it past college football. At some point, we were going to have to get jobs and start careers. It was a lot of pressure, but we had to pay the price if we wanted to play the game. In the same way, you must also pay the price if you want to stay focused on what you must do. A focused life involves a total dedication. You have to think of it like this: you can pay now, or you can pay later.

The truth is that here are no victories at bargain prices. As Proverbs 13:4 says, "The soul of a lazy man desires, and has nothing; but the soul of the diligent shall be made rich." Lazy people get nothing in the end! If you want to reach that endzone and win, you can't be lazy. You can desire it, talk about it and even write out a fabulous plan as to how you are going to achieve it, but if you don't do the hard work necessary to get you there, you might as well forget it. It's not going to happen. You won't win if you are still that lazy bum sitting in a La-Z-Boy. As I said before, there is no pill, potion or gadget for $19.99 that you can buy that will solve all your problems. You have to pay the price and work through the sweat and tears. The good news is that the reward is surely great!

Aim at Your Goals

Any athlete who trains in his or her sport understands what the goals are. A runner is focused on the finish line at the end of the race. A boxer is looking for that knockout punch that takes an opponent down. An offensive lineman is looking for the perfect opportunity to crush, stop and take out the target. The entire football team is focused on moving the ball down the field to their endzone to score the winning touchdown. They all know what their goals are.

The same applies to you when living a focused life. You have to identify the specific course or direction for your life—the vision for your future. Proverbs 29:18 puts it this way: "Where there is no vision, the people perish: but he that keepeth the law, happy is he" (*KJV*). Simply put, without a vision, plan or direction, you die!

Did that get your attention? If that doesn't wake you up, I don't know what will. It's critical that you set goals for the direction of your life and put an action plan together to achieve them. One of my favorite verses is Habakkuk 2:2, in which the Lord says, "Write the vision and make it plain on tablets, that he may run who reads it." This verse outlines such a simple method: write, run and read. Write the vision down so you know where you are going and how you are going to get there. Guys, you might not like to ask for directions, but you need to move in the right direction, and writing your goals down is a good place to start. At the end of this chapter, I will show you some ways for you to do this.

If you are feeling more than a little overwhelmed at this stage of the game, that's okay. Talk to your heavenly Coach, and ask Him to guide you, direct you and give you the wisdom you need to start making better choices. He will help you overcome the lies Satan has been using to keep you in bondage. Pray and ask God for help when writing your goals and plan, and then pray for the strength and determination to achieve them.

Stay in Control

The final strategy I want to give you before you walk out of our locker room is to stay in control. To do this, you will have to have complete discipline. Paul put it this way: "But I discipline my body and bring it into subjection, lest, when I have preached to others, I myself should become disqualified" (1 Corinthians 9:27). You have to keep your body in subjection in order to keep your focus. You have to discipline yourself to do the right thing all the time, because if you don't, you can become a castaway. There are rules in sports and rules in healthy living, and when you break the rules, you pay a price and run the risk of being disqualified.

During the Olympics in Seoul, Korea, in 1988, a sprinter from Canada named Ben Johnson became the fastest human being ever by running the 100 meters in 9.79 seconds. It was a great moment in Canadian sports, but just 62 hours later, Olympic officials walked into his room and took back his gold medal. Why? Because he had tested positive for steroids. He had broken the rules and had to be disqualified. He hadn't disciplined himself in the right way, and because he tried to take the fast-track to success, he went from hero to zero in only 62 hours.

Imagine reaching the pinnacle of your sports career only to lose it in matter of hours. This is why discipline is so important. Athletes have to be disciplined to tell their bodies no when the desire comes to put steroids or junk into it. They must say to themselves, *I am not going to do it*. Their focus is on living a disciplined life so they can win and win square and fair.

Now, guys, there is only one way to have self-control in your life, and that is through Spirit control. You need to be led and guided by the Holy Spirit. In Galatians 5:16, Paul says, "I say then: Walk in the Spirit, and you shall not fulfill the lust of the flesh." If you are Spirit-controlled, you won't want to give in to those fleshly desires. You won't want to be anywhere other than where God wants you to be. There is also power when the Spirit controls your life. I love what 1 John 4:4 has to say about this: "You are of God, little children, and have overcome them, because He who is in you is greater than he who is in the world." You are an overcomer when you are Spirit-controlled, and Satan has no power over you. You can be victorious.

The Most Important Play Is the Next Play

The last item I want to leave with you before we head out to the field is something my football coach at Liberty drilled into us players again and again: "The most important play is the next play." He was constantly telling us to forget about the past and what had just happened on the field. If we messed up and blew a play, it was done, and we needed to move on. If someone fumbled the ball or accidentally went offsides, we needed to learn from it and focus on what we are supposed to do next. If we missed a tackle, that was okay; just try not to do it again.

The coach's point was this: you can't focus on your past failures, because the most important play is coming up. It's what you do *next* that counts. I want to leave that same message with you: your most important play in this game of getting healthy is your next play. It's time to forget about your past mistakes and failures and focus on your next steps—your A.C.T.I.O.N. plan for getting in shape. Don't let the past cripple your future; learn from it and move on. Put all your time and energy into your *next* play.

You're ready for the big game now. I have faith in you. I know you can do it. So leave this locker room with your head held high, ready to take out anything that gets in your way. Oh, and by the way, that last game I played at Liberty on November 10, 1979, we beat Canisius College 17 to 10. So now it's your turn to go out there and win. Remember you only have one shot—one life—so don't waste it.

Thomas Vidaurri
Takes Action

LOST 166 POUNDS

Before	After
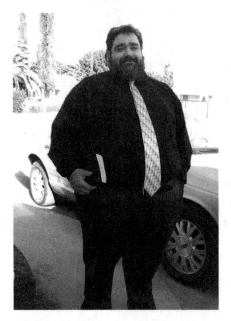	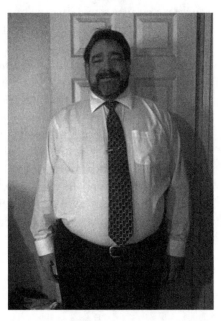

I have had a lifetime of struggling with weight issues, and along with the obesity came depression and chronic back and groin pain. Approximately seven years ago, I realized the first onset of symptoms from diabetes. After a couple more years of weight gain, I found myself in the hospital with severe morbid obesity. I weighed 500 pounds and had a BMI of 73.8 and a blood sugar level of 1,200. My doctor said I was a walking coma. I was immediately put on insulin injections.

Some years before, I had been diagnosed with high blood pressure and sleep apnea. I would stop breathing for up to a minute at a time. After I exhaled the oxygen from my system, I would gasp for another breath. Because of my weight, each and every breath was a near-death experience. After a couple more trips to the hospital for chest pains—which, praise

God, were not due to a heart attack but to a muscular-skeletal problem caused by my obesity—I was diagnosed with 89 percent stenosis in my left carotid artery. This is a narrowing of the main artery on the left side of the neck that carries blood to the brain.

I was so overweight that it was hard for me to walk from my couch to the mailbox. At times I did manage to go out with a church team for an hour or so to knock on doors and pass out tracts. Afterward, I would end up suffering and in pain. I would swell up and lie in bed for three or four days.

It seemed that my only option was to have bariatric surgery—a drastic surgery in which doctors restructure the stomach to approximately the size of an egg. I met all the criteria for the surgery, so I took some classes for six months, met with doctors and psychiatrists, and prepared to have the procedure done the following year. But I didn't go through with it. In fact, I actually repeated the pre-surgery procedure three years in a row, but God intervened and kept me from going ahead with it. God had something better for me. In Matthew 6:33, Jesus says, "But seek first the kingdom of God and His righteousness, and all these things shall be added to you." What are the "all these things" that will be added? They are His grace and mercy, better health, and a more abundant and fulfilling life.

My pastor, Karsten Polk, and I had been praying about my weight loss. I remember he even fasted with me for about a week as I detoxified my system with an herbal fiber blend. This was just before he purchased Pastor Steve's book *Bod4God: The Four Keys to Weight Loss*. I read the book and started applying the basic principles that Pastor Steve had laid out. I finally realized I was tired of living life like this and depriving my wife, my family, and myself of the abundant life that God can give.

I took to heart a foundational idea in the book that shed a new light on weight loss: that of applying biblical principles to my problem. Paul's words in 1 Corinthians 6:19-20 made a huge difference in the way I viewed my problem: "Do you not know that your body is the temple of the Holy Spirit who is in you, whom you have from God, and you are not your own? For you were bought at a price; therefore glorify God in your body and in your spirit, which are God's." I began to understand that I needed to honor my body, for it is the Temple of the Holy Spirit. It was then and there that I put my all on the altar. I had tried many diets in the past, but I had never really given my weight problem to God.

I started my lifestyle change by cutting out all soft drinks and instead drinking up to a gallon of water a day. This alone made a huge difference. The next lifestyle change was to stop eating all fast food, which was followed by cutting my portion sizes. Over the next several months I saw some weight loss, but I had cut my calorie intake to the point I was starving myself. I figured that if I did not take in the calories, I could not possibly put on any more weight, and I would lose weight. That might have been true temporarily, but it was not a very healthy plan in the long run.

Since that time I have learned how to manage by food intake and incorporate exercise into my life. So far, I have lost a total of 166 pounds. My BMI is now 49.3—which is still high considering the recommended BMI is 30 or below. But praise God, my pants size has gone down from a 68 to a 48! I went from using insulin injections to treat my diabetes to several years of medications in pill form to requiring no diabetes medication. My average blood sugar currently runs about 87 to 90 before meals, which is right where it should be. The stenosis in my left carotid artery went from 89 percent to between 0 and 15 percent, which is a normal reading. I asked the doctors to explain how this could have happened. They could not, but I can: God still performs miracles today.

When I started the program, I had 36 percent lean body mass, which is the weight of everything in your body besides fat (muscle, organs, blood, bones and tissue). I had 47 percent "excess" weight, which is fat. When I finished the program, I had 57 percent lean body mass and 26 percent excess.

My current weight is 334 pounds. I want to lose at least another 100 pounds, and maybe a little more. Pastor Polk has been so inspired by my commitment and the transformation that has taken place in my life that this year he wants me to start a weight-loss class based on *Bod4God* and its biblical principles. When I contacted Pastor Reynolds, he was also so inspired by the many great accomplishments in my story that he said he would love to come to California to kick off our Losing to Live weight-loss competition.

I occasionally have the opportunity to preach to our congregation at Highland Baptist Temple. I used to get winded when I preached, but not any more. I am on fire for the Lord, and I see the work of the Holy Spirit exuding through me. I praise God for all that He has done for me and all that He is going to do through me. He not only saved my soul from hell but has also given me a rewarding, fulfilling, abundant and healthier life. Now I can serve Him with great energy, for "I can do all things through Christ who strengthens me" (Philippians 4:13).

Man Up

Eat Up: Green Up

Real men eat salad! Fill your salad with dark leafy greens such as spinach, romaine and leaf lettuces, which have been shown to protect against cancer, diabetes, heart disease, stroke and dementia. Vegetables are full of minerals, vitamins, enzymes and antioxidants that will energize you for living, and the more vegetables you eat, the more you lose! Just don't sabotage your salad by drowning it in dressing. Instead, put it on the side and dip your fork in before each bite. Vinaigrette-type dressings tend to have the lowest fat and sugar content.

Pump Up: Shadow Boom Boxing

For this exercise, put on your favorite song, bounce around, and throw some jabs, uppercuts and any punch combo that comes to mind. Challenge yourself to shadow box for the length of the song. Pretend you are in a ring fighting against the fat enemy. A song usually lasts for three minutes, so this intense cardio workout will challenge you both physically and mentally. Go until you have to throw in the towel!

A Final Word from Steve Reynolds

I firmly believe that any man's finest hour, the greatest fulfillment of all that he holds dear, is the moment when he has worked his heart out in a good cause and lies exhausted on the field of battle— victorious.

VINCE LOMBARDI

I hope you are pumped up, motivated and ready to move in the right direction. In this final section, instead of asking you some specific discussion questions, I want you to reflect on and discuss some of the principles we talked about in chapter 12. Basically, in order to stay focused, you need to (1) run to win, (2) pay the price, (3) aim at your goals and (4) stay in control. I've shared everything I can with you so you can win and be successful in getting healthier and in shape—it's all on you at this point. It's time for you to put it into practice and start working it out in your life, play by play. The best place to start is with your A.C.T.I.O.N. plan, so let's review what each of the steps in this acronym means.

Your A.C.T.I.O.N. Plan

Aware: Be *aware* of the seriousness of your physical condition and understand that your body matters to God.

Commit: *Commit* to living a disciplined life and to winning over temptation.

Transform: *Transform* the way you think and the way you live.

Incorporate: *Incorporate* healthy eating habits and exercise into your daily life.

Organize: *Organize* a team of people to help you win.

Navigate: Create an A.C.T.I.O.N. plan for healthy living so you can *navigate* your way to leaving a lasting legacy.

In the next two pages, I want you to sign the My Get Off the Couch Contract and write out your own A.C.T.I.O.N. plan for how you are going to get off the couch and get into shape. Hopefully, after reading each chapter, you have been writing down specific steps you can implement, and you can use this plan to organize all of those steps in one place. Keep your A.C.T.I.O.N. plan handy and visible so you can review it often, and don't forget to chart your progress. Writing items down will solidify them in your mind and help you stay on track. Don't be afraid to modify the list as things change in your life or if you find certain things are not working for you.

Once you have signed the contract and started working on your A.C.T.I.O.N. plan, share these vital steps and actions with your spouse, a friend, your team that you have been organizing, or your small group. Open up and share with others how strongly you feel about making this commitment and how you are going to need their support, encouragement and prayer as you start implementing these changes into your life. Ask them to walk alongside you as you navigate your way to living a healthier life, and give them permission to check on your progress. Remember that your goal is *progress*, not *perfection*. Just keep moving forward, slow and steady.

My Get Off the Couch Contract

It's time for some **A.C.T.I.O.N**. Now that you have read this book and are fully convinced you need to get off the couch and get into shape, it's time to make a commitment to get up and get moving.

Aware: I WILL be *aware* of the seriousness of my physical condition and understand that my body matters to God.

Commit: I WILL *commit* to living a disciplined life and to winning over temptation.

Transform: I WILL *transform* the way I think and the way I live.

Incorporate: I WILL *incorporate* healthy eating habits and exercise into my daily life.

Organize: I WILL *organize* a team of people to help me win.

Navigate: I WILL create an A.C.T.I.O.N. plan for healthy living so I can *navigate* my way to leaving a lasting legacy.

Knowing that my body is made by God and for God, I commit myself to getting off the couch and to leading a healthy lifestyle.

Name: _____ Date: _____

My A.C.T.I.O.N. Plan

Name: _____ Start Date: _____

My Short-term Goals: _____

My Long–term Goals: _____

Small Steps to Achieving These Goals

ACTION AND DESCRIPTION	START DATE	END DATE	ADDITIONAL COMMENTS
Aware			
Commit			
Transform			
Incorporate			
Organize			
Navigate			

My Progress Report

In order to know what progress you are making, you need a place to record where you began and whether you are losing or gaining weight. Please fill out the information requested below. Each week for 12 weeks, record your progress. It's important, so be faithful to record your progress.

Name: _____ Start Date: _____ End Date: _____

My Starting Weight: _____ My Final Weight: _____

Goal: _____

My Starting Measurements:

Neck: _____

Arm (Bicep): _____

Chest: _____

Waist: _____

Hips: _____

Thighs: _____

Calf: _____

My Ending Measurements:

Neck: _____

Arm (Bicep): _____

Chest: _____

Waist: _____

Hips: _____

Thighs: _____

Calf: _____

My Weight Loss

Week	+ / -	Week	+ / -
1		7	
2		8	
3		9	
4		10	
5		11	
6		12	

The Top Five Health Numbers to Know

As I mentioned in this book, some guys know every sports statistic there is to know, but most of those same guys wouldn't have a clue about the numbers related to their health—the numbers that mean life or death to them. Here is a quick list of the five most important health numbers you should know.

1. Waist Size

If you can only remember one number, remember your waist size because it is a better predictor of your risk of heart disease than just your weight or your BMI (see item 2). An expanded waist size of more than 40 inches increases your risk of cardiovascular disease, diabetes, metabolic problems, high blood pressure and abnormal cholesterol. Belly fat sends out a toxic stream of chemicals that will impact your entire body.

How to Measure Waist Size
Use a piece of non-stretch tape and measure one-inch above your belly button, not where your belt lies or around your hips. This is your natural waistline and is just above your hipbone and below the ribcage. Stand up tall and suck in your stomach (spare tire). The fat you're measuring is deep inside the belly.

What Your Waist Measurement Should Be
In men, the waist size should be less than 40 inches. The ideal number is 35 inches.

2. Weight and Body Measurement Index (BMI)

BMI is a measure of body fat based on height and weight that applies to both adult men and women. To determine this number, weigh in at least once a week, and try to do so first thing in the morning. If you weigh frequently, remember that it is common to have daily fluctuations in weight.

How to Calculate Your BMI
1. Weigh yourself first thing in the morning, without clothes.
2. Measure your height in inches.
3. Multiply your weight in pounds by 700.
4. Divide the answer in #3 by your height.
5. Divide the answer in #4 by your height again.
6. The answer in #5 is your BMI.

What Your BMI Should Be
If the number you obtain is 25 to 29.9, you are considered *overweight*. If the number is 30 or higher, you are considered *obese*. Note that BMI alone may overestimate obesity, so some health care providers recommend using BMI in combination with a waist-to-hip ratio (which is another indicator of belly fat). To get this number, measure your waist one-inch above the belly button and your hips at the greatest measurement (thigh bone socket). For men, an optimal waist-to-hip ratio is <.9.

3. Cholesterol (Both Good and Bad)

Cholesterol isn't all bad, but, as you've probably heard, there is "good" (HDL) cholesterol and "bad" (LDL) cholesterol.

How to Remember the Difference Between HDL and LDL
Here's a way to remember the difference: good cholesterol is the "**H**appy" kind, with an *H;* while LDL cholesterol is the "**L**ousy" kind, with an *L.* The blood tests needed to determine the levels of each of these kinds of cholesterol will also give you a triglyceride reading. All three scores are important.

Numbers to Strive For
Total cholesterol: you want a number of 200 or lower.
HDL: You want to see a number of 40 or higher.
LDL: The optimal level is 100 or lower. If you have other major risk factors, such as pre-existing cardiovascular disease or diabetes, your doctor may want your LDL closer to 70.
Triglycerides: You want to see a number of less than 150.

4. Blood Pressure

One in three adults in the U.S. has high blood pressure or pre-hypertension. According to the American Heart Association, from 1996 to 2006, the number of deaths from high blood pressure rose by more than 48 percent.[1]

Your *systolic* (top) measurement indicates the pressure of blood against artery walls when the heart pumps blood out during a heartbeat, while the *diastolic* (bottom) measurement indicates the same pressure between heartbeats, when the heart fills with blood. Both of these numbers are important. Hypertension (high blood pressure) occurs when systolic blood pressure is 140 or higher and diastolic pressure is 90 or higher.

What Your Numbers Should Be

Your top (systolic) blood pressure number should be less than 120.
Your bottom (diastolic) number should be less than 80.
The ideal blood pressure is approximately 115 over 75.

How to Check Your Own Blood Pressure

Visit your local pharmacy and use their machine, or invest in a device you can use at home and learn how to test your own blood pressure. For accuracy, take three readings and figure out the average.

When to Check Your Blood Pressure

If you are overweight and/or at risk, check your blood pressure once a month. Make sure you are testing at the same point in the day, when you're most relaxed. A systolic reading above 140 is considered too high and warrants seeing your doctor.

5. Fasting Blood Sugar

A blood sugar reading indicates the amount of glucose (sugar) present in the blood. Being overweight and/or inactive can increase your risk of developing type 2 diabetes, a condition in which the body does not produce enough of a chemical called *insulin* to allow glucose (the primary source of energy for the body) into the cells.

How to Check Your Blood Sugar Levels

Your blood sugar levels will need to be determined by blood tests your doctor orders. Take these tests eight hours after your last food intake. If you become a type 2 diabetic, you will likely get a blood glucose monitor and a schedule for testing yourself.

What Your Numbers Should Be

Your fasting glucose level should be less than 100. A more definitive measurement of blood sugar levels can be determined through an A1C test, which indicates glucose levels over a three-month span. Using this test, you may be *pre-diabetic* if your fasting blood sugar is 100 to 125, or if you have an A1C of 5.7 percent to 6.4 percent. You may be *diabetic* if your fasting blood sugar is 126 or greater, or if you have an A1C of 6.5 percent (and you've received) these results two or more times. Doctors like to see a level of 7 percent or less on an A1C test.

How to Find a Personal Trainer

You know how it is: you walk into a workout facility and look around, and there are two-dozen different kinds of machines you could use. You have no clue what they are for, how to get the maximum benefit from them, and how to avoid injury while using them. The best way to resolve this dilemma is by hiring a personal trainer, who can guide you in the use of the machines and other activities to maximize the value you will receive from them. But how do you find a personal trainer? How do you find a personal trainer who fits you and your needs? Most workout facilities have a trainer on staff. Some are great, some are good, and some are mediocre. In addition, some of the great ones are great for another client, but not for you. So, how do you find the right match?

Tips for Picking a Trainer

You want to pick a trainer in much the same way as you would hire an employee for your company, or buy a new car, or pick a wife. Although "picking a wife" might seem a bit extreme, in some ways it is the most appropriate comparison, as you will be spending a great deal of time with the trainer. So a good fit is important. Given this, here are a few questions to ask yourself to help you pick the right trainer.

- Is the facility clean?
- Are the machines in good working order?
- Does the facility have trainers on staff?
- What are the trainer's credentials?
- With whom is he or she certified?
- Are the credentials current?
- How long has he or she been training?
- What kind of training is his or her expertise?

- Does that fit with your goals?
- What success has the trainer had with his or her clients?
- Can you interview some of them?
- What is the person's style of training? (Aggressive? Encouraging?)
- How much does the trainer charge?
- Does he or she offer small-group sessions or online training?

After you choose a trainer—but before you begin working with him or her—list your goals. Where do you want to be in six months from now? In a year? Make sure the plan the trainer describes includes exercises to work your upper body, your lower body, and any problem areas you need to have included.

Show Up

During your first few sessions, decide how well the two of you sync. Do you understand what he or she is telling you to do? Is the trainer listening to your concerns and answering your questions? A good trainer will want to equip you for a lifetime of healthy living and will be willing to answer your questions and guide you into the best workout routine.

Show up for the first session ready to work. Don't waste the trainer's time and your time and money—he or she will get paid even if you don't show. Be honest about any injuries you might have. If a previous workout has left you in pain, tell the trainer right away. He or she will know how to help you work through and around these kinds of problems.

Ending the Training Relationship

All training relationships come to an end. If your trainer has been working with you to overcome surgery or an injury, when you get better, you are done. If your goal was to lose weight and you have, it's probably time to move into maintenance mode. Get some final help from the trainer about how to continue doing some of the exercises at home. Get a plan for going on with the good things that have been happening in your life as a result of working with a trainer. If you and your trainer have disagreed, or if you don't believe things are working out for you the way you had hoped, be honest with your trainer and tell him or her you will be moving on and why.

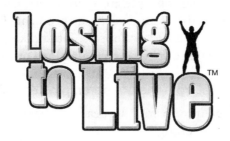

How to Set Up a Losing to Live Competition

Can individuals lose weight without being believers—without God? Can they lose weight without a competition? Yes, they can, but it is our experience that people do best when they first commit their weight problem to God and then ask for His help on a daily basis. They also do well when they are part of a competition in which they are encouraged by others to take those steps that will help them lose weight. I believe with all my heart that a competition is essential to weight loss. We all need connection and a place to share our successes and failures. So don't try to lose weight alone—join a team of losers!

Here is a simple guide for setting up a Losing to Live weight-loss competition. For more information than is given here, purchase a Losing to Live Group Starter Kit (available at **www.bod4god.org**). This kit contains the following:

- *Bod4God: The Four Keys to Weight Loss* by Steve Reynolds, which provides additional details on how to set up a group competition.
- The *Bod4God* DVD series, which includes group starter tools.
- A Losing to Live T-shirt.
- A Losing to Live magnet.

What to Do Before the Competition

Step 1: Know Your Purposes

If you are clear about your purposes and can articulate them to a pastor, to key leaders and to a congregation, you will quickly gain their approval. Christians are the most overweight people group in America, and Losing to Live has been designed to confront and solve this problem. This program will show people in your church how to lose weight and keep it off through a Bod4God lifestyle. The bottom line is changing lives one pound at a time.

Step 2: Seek Approval from the Leadership of Your Church

- If you are the *pastor*, inform your key leaders what you are planning to do and why you are doing it.

- If you are *not the pastor*, go first to your pastor and share your passion to help church members to lose weight. Let the pastor inform the key leaders.

- Tell all those in leadership what the program will cost the church in terms of dollars for advertising, purchasing the participant kits (if the church is going to provide any of the kits for participants—see step 9), coffee, snacks or lunches and any other expenses you foresee. Tell the leadership how you plan to fund the program (for example, through offerings, registration fees or fundraisers).

Step 3: Establish Your Location

The entire competition takes 12 weeks. Participants meet once a week for 90 minutes. During the first 30 minutes everyone will meet together to hear overall results and listen to a speaker. During the remaining 60 minutes, participants will break into teams for discussion. Keeping this in mind, you will need:

- A place large enough for all participants to meet together such as an auditorium, multipurpose room, or fellowship hall.
- Smaller rooms where individual teams can meet.
- A private place to put your scale for weigh-ins.

Step 4: Determine Your Schedule

The group in our church meets on Sunday nights from 6:00 to 7:30 PM. You can meet any time that works best for your church or organization. Remember that the total time for a meeting is 90 minutes, which includes 30 minutes for the total group rally time and 60 minutes for the small-group time.

Step 5: Recruit and Assign Leaders

You will need a director, team captains and administrative support to do the weigh-ins and other activities during the sessions. Think long and pray earnestly about who these people should be, as they will be crucial to the success of the program. Specifically, seek out those who will be able to:

- *Educate the participants.* These people may include doctors, nutritionists, physical coaches and others in your congregation with certain areas of expertise.

- *Encourage the participants through worship and devotional times.* These people may include those who have themselves lost weight and know how long and difficult the process can be.

- *Equip the participants.* Look for people who can help train the participants with regard to eating healthy and exercising. Look around, and you will be sure to find someone who is leading a Pilates or aerobics class or who is known for his or her healthy cooking. Press them into service for this program.

Step 6: Organize Your Registration Process

All participants must fill out a Losing to Live registration form (this is part of the *Bod4God* DVD series in the Losing to Live Group Starter Kit). Collect these well in advance of the competition. (You will need this information to properly order your participant kits.)

Step 7: Implement Your Promotion Strategy

Your promotion should target your church and community. A promotional video and other materials are included in the *Bod4God* DVD series.

Step 8: Host an Orientation Meeting

Two to three weeks before the first competition, host an orientation meeting for potential participants. The goal is to explain how it works and then register participants for the upcoming 12-week competition. Distribute the Losing to Live Fact Sheet and show the orientation video presentation by Pastor Steve Reynolds, both of which are part of the *Bod4God* DVD series.

Step 9: Order Your Participant Kits

I recommend that each participant obtain an official Losing to Live Participant Kit (available at www.bod4god.org), which contains *Bod4God: Four Keys to Weight Loss*. Each participant will need a book to do the Victory

Guide exercises and other exercises that are crucial elements to success in the program. Also included is an official Losing to Live T-shirt and a refrigerator magnet.

Step 10: Determine Your Teams
After each participant has been registered, divide the enrollees into teams of 6 to 12 people. Each team should be balanced out between those who need to lose a lot of weight and those who need to lose less weight. Don't worry if you have only one or two teams the first time. As these first teams have success, others will notice and join the program.

Step 11: Set Up Your Weigh-in Procedure
You will need a good-quality scale and a private place for the weigh-in—setting up the scale in a classroom is often ideal. Have participants come in one at a time to weigh in so as to respect their privacy. For the convenience of participants, you may want to schedule several weigh-in times. The weight-loss competition is based on the percentage of weight loss, not the amount of weight loss. Most groups use a Microsoft Office Excel spreadsheet to do their calculations (you can also have participants use the My Progress Report in appendix A).

Step 12: Set Up How You Will Communicate with Participants
Get email addresses and phone numbers from all participants. For the best success, the director and the group leaders need to be in contact with the participants on a weekly basis. (A few "atta boys" will encourage participants to stay on track.)

What to Do During the Competition

Step 1: Conduct Weekly Weigh-ins
Schedule specific times the participants can weigh in. These might be in conjunction with a Sunday morning church service or your weekly rally time. Record the participant's weight each week without comment. Whether they have lost or gained weight, this is their story to tell. Say nothing to the participant or anyone else.

Step 2: Conduct Weekly Rally Time
At the rally, announce individual teams' total weight loss. Individuals will also be competing to be one of the top 10 losers of the 12-week competition. Also, line up a speaker for each rally. Have an "expert" speak about ex-

ercise, nutrition or attitude. These individuals can come either from your congregation or from outside your church. Another option to having live speakers is to use the videos in the *Bod4God* DVD series. These videos are designed to be a perfect complement to *Bod4God*.

Step 3: Conduct Weekly Small Groups

Small groups will meet following the weekly rally time. Most participants will connect best with the program in their small group teams. Each team should choose a team name based on a fruit or vegetable as a rallying cry. During each team meeting, the participants should:

- Go over the information in *Bod4God* chapter by chapter
- Specifically discuss the weekly Victory Guide assignments (found at the end of each chapter in *Bod4God*)
- Share ideas on what works and what doesn't work for each person
- Cheer each other's successes
- Pray with each other

Step 4: Conduct a Victory Celebration

Although the weekly rally time is a kind of celebration, you want to have a big final rally celebratory event. Note that:

- During this last-week celebration, you will change the order of the meeting by having the small group time first and the rally time second. (The small groups will meet first to go over the material in week 12 in *Bod4God*.)
- You will announce the overall weight loss for the group and the various teams during the celebration and recognize the individual biggest loser(s). Give each participant a certificate of participation found in the *Bod4God* DVD series including group starter tools (available at www.bod4god.org).
- You should decide if you would like to give out prizes.
- Any food for this event should be healthy.
- If you have individuals who have had unusual success, you may want to call in the media to do a story.
- You will want to rejoice over what God has helped you accomplish together. Make sure everyone leaves feeling like a winner.
- Announce your next competition.

Get Off the Couch
Key Bible Verses

*Then Jesus said to those Jews who believed Him, "If you
abide in My word, you are My disciples indeed. And you shall
know the truth, and the truth shall make you free."*
JOHN 8:31-32

As I have stated throughout this book, the Bible is absolute truth. Jesus
said that by knowing the truth, we can be set free from sin. The battle to
get off the couch and get into shape will be won or lost in the mind, so fill
your mind with the Word of God.

There are 12 keys verses used in *Get Off the Couch* that reinforce each action step, each of which appears on the following page. I recommend mem-
orizing one verse each week if possible, as they will encourage you to stay
true to your goal of leading a healthier life. Copy the verse on a card each
week and post it in your car, on your bathroom mirror, on your computer
screen or anywhere else where you will see it first thing in the morning.

Aware

Philippians 4:13: "I can do all things through Christ who strengthens me."

1 Corinthians 6:19: "Do you not know that your body is the temple of the Holy Spirit who is in you, whom you have from God, and you are not your own?"

Commit

Proverbs 3:7-8: "Do not be wise in your own eyes; fear the LORD and depart from evil. It will be health to your flesh, and strength to your bones."

Matthew 26:41: "Watch and pray, lest you enter into temptation."

Transform

Romans 8:5: "For those who live according to the flesh set their minds on the things of the flesh, but those who live according to the Spirit, the things of the Spirit."

Hebrews 12:1: "Therefore we also, since we are surrounded by so great a cloud of witnesses, let us lay aside every weight, and the sin which so easily ensnares us, and let us run with endurance the race that is set before us."

Incorporate

Proverbs 23:2: "And put a knife to your throat if you are a man given to appetite."

Isaiah 40:31: "But those who wait on the LORD shall renew their strength; they shall mount up with wings like eagles, they shall run and not be weary, they shall walk and not faint."

Organize

Ecclesiastes 4:12: "Though one may be overpowered by another, two can withstand him. And a threefold cord is not quickly broken."

Proverbs 27:17: "As iron sharpens iron, so a man sharpens the countenance of his friend."

Navigate

2 Timothy 4:7: "I have fought the good fight, I have finished the race, I have kept the faith."

Habakkuk 2:2: "Then the LORD answered me and said: 'Write the vision and make it plain on tablets, that he may run who reads it.'"

Endnotes

Introduction: A Man's A.C.T.I.O.N. Plan
1. The Man Up/Check Up sidebars were contributed by Nigel M. Azer, MD.

Chapter 1: Get in the Game
1. "Obesity: Unhealthy and Unmanly," *Harvard Men's Health Watch,* March 2011. http://www.health.harvard.edu/newsletters/Harvard_Mens_Health_Watch/2011/March/obesity-unhealthy-and-unmanly.
2. G. Corona, E. Mannucci, A.D. Fisher, et al., "Low Levels of Androgens in Men with Erectile Dysfunction and Obesity," *Journal of Sexual Medicine,* 2008, vol. 5, pp. 2454-2463.
3. Steve Reynolds's book *Bod4God: The Four Keys to Weight Loss* (Ventura, CA: Regal, 2009), is available at www,amazon.com, www.barnesandnoble.com, and retailers nationwide. For more information, see www.regalbooks.com and www.bod4god.org.

Chapter 2: Your Body Matters to God
1. Joe Gibbs, "Two Minute Drill: Be Nice to Your Body," Crosswalk.com, March 12. http://www.crosswalk.com/devotionals/two-minute-drills/two-minute-drill-week-of-march-12.html.
2. "Clinical Guidelines on the Identification, Evaluation, and Treatment of Overweight and Obesity in Adults: Executive Summary," National Institutes of Health, National Heart, Lung, and Blood Institute, June 1998.
3. "Overweight and Obesity: A Major Public Health Issue," U.S. Department of Health and Human Services Prevention Report, 2001, vol. 16, no. 1.
4. Heather M. Brinson, "The Human Body—Wired for Extremes: True Stories of Survival," Answers in Genesis, September 1, 2009. http://www.answersingenesis.org/articles/am/v4/n4/wired-for-extremes.
5. Michael Matthews, "Wonders of the Human Body," Answers in Genesis, September 20, 2009. http://www.answersingenesis.org/articles/2009/09/20/human-body-promo
6. Ibid.
7. David Menton, Ph.D., "The Amazing Human Hair," Answers in Genesis, July 4, 2007. http://www.answersingenesis.org/articles/am/v2/n3/amazing-human-hair.
8. David Demick, "The Breath of Life: God's Gift to All Creatures," Answers in Genesis, December 1, 2004. http://www.answersingenesis.org/articles/cm/v27/n1/breath-of-life.
9. Ibid.
10. David Menton, Ph.D., "The Hearing Ear," Answers in Genesis, August 29, 2007. http://www.answersingenesis.org/articles/am/v2/n4/hearing-ear.

Chapter 3: You Gotta Play by the Playbook
1. Elizabeth Merrill, "In NFL, the Playbook Is Sacred," ESPN.com, August 29, 2007. http://sports.espn.go.com/nfl/preview07/news/story?id=2973338.
2. R.C. Whitaker, J.A. Wright, M.S. Pepe, et al., "Predicting Obesity in Young Adulthood from Childhood and Parental Obesity," *The New England Journal of Medicine,* September 25, 1997, vol. 337, no. 13, pp. 869-873.

Chapter 4: Winning Over Temptation
1. M. Sullivan, J. Karlsson, L. Sjöström, et al., "Swedish Obese Subjects (SOS)—An Intervention Study of Obesity: Baseline Evaluation of Health and Psychosocial Functioning in the First 1743 Subjects Examined," *International Journal of Obesity and Related Metabolic Disorders,* September 1993, vol. 17, pp. 503-512.

Chapter 5: Get Your Head in the Game

1. The following is from a personal interview with the author.
2. John Cawley and Chad Meyerhoefer, "The Medical Care Costs of Obesity: An Instrumental Variables Approach," *Journal of Health Economics*, 2012, vol. 31, issue 1, pp. 219-230.

Chapter 6: Progress, Not Perfection

1. For you sports fans, they are: (1) Frank Filchock to Andy Farkas (Washington Redskins, 1939); (2) George Izo to Bobby Mitchell (Washington Redskins, 1963); (3) Karl Sweetan to Pat Studstill (Detroit Lions, 1966); (4) Sonny Jurgensen to Jerry Allen (Washington Redskins, 1968); (5) Jim Plunkett to Cliff Branch (Los Angeles Raiders, 1983); (6) Ron Jaworski to Mike Quick (Philadelphia Eagles, 1985); (7) Stan Humphries to Tony Martin (San Diego Chargers, 1994); (8) Brett Favre to Robert Brooks (Green Bay Packers, 1995); (9) Trent Green to Marc Boerigter (Kansas City Chiefs, 2002); (10) Jeff Garcia to Andre Davis (Cleveland Browns, 2004); (11) Gus Frerotte to Bernard Berrian (Minnesota Vikings, 2008); (12) Tom Brady to Wes Welker (New England Patriots, 2011); (13) Eli Manning to Victor Cruz (New York Giants, 2011). See "99-Yard Pass Play," Wikipedia.org. http://en.wikipedia.org/wiki/99-yard_pass_play.

Chapter 7: Get Buff, *Not* Buffeted

1. Bill Liggett, "When the California Fast-food Chain In-N-Out Opened Three New Restaurants in and Around Dallas, Texas, Recently, Chaos Ensued," *The Herald Sun,* June 2011. http://www.heraldsun.com/view/full_story/14470480/article-When-the-California-fast-food-chain-In-N-Out-opened-three-new-restaurants-in-and-around-Dallas—Texas—recently—chaos-ensued.
2. "Sports Nutrition," The University of Nebraska, 2012. http://www.huskers.com/ViewArticle.dbml?DB_OEM_ID=100&ATCLID=1552880.
3. E.E. Calle, M.J. Thun, J.M. Petrelli, et al., "Body-Mass Index and Mortality in a Prospective Cohort of U.S. Adults," *New England Journal of Medicine,* October 7, 1999, vol. 341, pp. 1097-1141.
4. Shereen Jegtiv, "You Need to Drink More Water," About.com Nutrition, July 22, 2012. http://nutrition.about.com/od/hydrationwater/a/waterarticle.htm.
5. "Symptoms of Dehydration," The Mayo Clinic, January 7, 2011. http://www.mayoclinic.com/health/dehydration/DS00561/DSECTION=symptoms.
6. Michele Stanton, *Prevention's Firm Up in 3 Weeks: Trim and Tone Your Trouble Zones for Your Best Body Ever* (New York: Rodale Books, 2004), p. 33.
7. Elaine Magee, MPH, RD, "Choosing a Healthy Breakfast Cereal," MedicineNet.com, July 3, 2007. http://www.medicinenet.com/script/main/art.asp?articlekey=82374&page=2.
8. "Fair Packaging and Labeling Act (US)," 15 USC 1451-1461, Wikipedia.org. http://en.wikipedia.org/wiki/Fair_Packaging_and_Labeling_Act_%28US%29.
9. J.M. Andrews, "How Much Protein Does the Average Man Need?" LiveStrong.com, April 22, 2011. http://www.livestrong.com/article/425810-how-much-protein-does-the-average-man-need/.
10. If figuring out nutrition labels doesn't come easily to you, visit the Mayo Clinic website for an interactive label. When you hover your cursor over certain portions of the label, you will find good information on which nutrients you should try to increase and which you should avoid. See http://www.mayoclinic.com/health/nutrition-facts/NU00293.
11. "Choosing Healthy Fats: Good Fats, Bad Fats, and the Power of Omega-3S," HelpGuide.org. http://www.helpguide.org/life/healthy_diet_fats.htm.
12. "Walter Willett: The Professor Who Saw the Light," Stop Trans Fats. http://www.stop-trans-fat.com/walter-willett.html.
13. "Four Most Harmful Ingredients in Packaged Foods," Reader's Digest. http://www.rd.com/health/diet-weight-loss/4-most-harmful-ingredients-in-packaged-foods/.
14. Ibid.
15. Nanci Hellmich, "Bread Is a Big Source of Americans' Salt Intake, Too," *USA Today,* March 5, 2012. http://www.usatoday.com/news/health/story/health/story/2012-03-04/Bread-is-a-big-source-of-Americans-salt-intake-too/53357294/1.
16. "Four Most Harmful Ingredients in Packaged Foods," Reader's Digest.
17. Ibid.

Chapter 8: No Pain, No Gain!

1. Michele Stanton, *Prevention's Firm Up in 3 Weeks: Trim and Tone Your Trouble Zones for Your Best Body Ever* (New York: Rodale Books, 2004), p. 6.
2. James A. Levine, MD, PhD, "What Are the Risks of Sitting Too Much?" The Mayo Clinic. http://www.mayoclinic.com/health/sitting/AN02082.
3. Daryl Laws, "For Many of Us, Sitting Has Become the New 'Smoking.'" The Times News, January 2, 2012. http://www.thetimesnews.com/articles/body-51071-fitness-work.html.
4. The Greek word translated as "carpenter" in Matthew 13:55 and Mark 6:3 is *tekton*, which is a general word that referred to maker of objects of various materials (even a builder). However, Jesus' association with being a carpenter appears in early Christian tradition and in the writings of Justin Martyr (d. ad 165), who said he was a maker of yokes and ploughs. Regardless, the word implies that Joseph and Jesus were involved in manual labor.
5. D.A. Katz, C.A. McHomey and R.L. Atkinson, "Impact of Obesity on Health-Related Quality of Life in Patients with Chronic Illness," *Journal of General Internal Medicine*, November 2000, vol. 15, no. 11, pp. 789-796.
6. Martin Chase, "NFL Training Camp—This Is Where Football Begins," StreetDirectory.com. http://www.streetdirectory.com/travel_guide/46337/recreation_and_sports/nfl_training_camp_this_is_where_football_begins.html.
7. Betsy Noxon, "Want to Lose Weight? Get Some Sleep," *US News & World Report*, May 25, 2012. http://health.usnews.com/health-news/articles/2012/05/25/want-to-lose-weight-get-some-sleep.
8. Madison Park, "Why We're Sleeping Less," data from annual Sleep in America Poll, CNN, March 4, 2009. http://articles.cnn.com/2009-03-04/health/sleep.stress.economy_1_national-sleep-foundation-poll-anxiety?_s=PM:HEALTH.
9. Dr. Michael Breus, quoted in Denise Mann, "Sleep and Weight Gain: Will Better Sleep Help You Avoid Extra Pounds?" http://www.webmd.com/sleep-disorders/excessive-sleepiness-10/lack-of-sleep-weight-gain.
10. Orfeu Buxton, quoted in Noxon, "Want to Lose Weight? Get Some Sleep."
11. Brueus, quoted in Mann, "Sleep and Weight Gain: Will Better Sleep Help You Avoid Extra Pounds?"
12. Plamen Penev, MD, PhD, et al, "Cutting Back on Sleep Reduces the Benefits of Dieting," *ScienceDaily*, October 2, 2010. http://www.sciencedaily.com/releases/2010/10/101004211637.htm.
13. Jerry Kram, quoted in Noxon, "Want to Lose Weight? Get Some Sleep."
14. James K. Wyatt, PhD, quoted in Sari Harrar, "Solved—Your Personal Energy Crisis," *Good Housekeeping*. http://www.goodhousekeeping.com/health/wellness/morning-caffeine#slide-4.
15. Joy Bauer, "Can't Sleep? Change Your Diet," *TODAY*, April 18, 2007. http://today.msnbc.msn.com/id/18043086/ns/today-today_health/t/cant-sleep-change-your-diet/#.UDaRtES2I7C.
16. Lindsay Lyon, "10 Ways to Get Better Sleep (and Maybe Cure Your Insomnia)," *US News & World Report*. http://health.usnews.com/health-news/family-health/slideshows/sleep-better/2.
17. Matt Fitzgerald, "Quick-Start Fitness: A Beginner's Guide," Experience Life, January-February 2008. http://experiencelife.com/article/quick-start-fitness-a-beginners-guide/.
18. "Exercise: 7 Benefits of Regular Physical Activity," The Mayo Clinic. http://www.mayoclinic.com/health/exercise/HQ01676/NSECTIONGROUP=2.
19. Winston Churchill, speech at Harrow School in London, England, October 29, 1941.

Chapter 9: Stronger Together

1. David A. Beuther, Scott T. Weiss and E. Rand Sutherland, "Obesity and Asthma," *American Journal of Respiratory and Critical Care Medicine*, July 15, 2006, vol. 174, pp. 112-119.
2. Denise Mann, "Want to Lose Weight? Try Teamwork," WebMD, February 17, 2012, http://www.webmd.com/diet/news/20120217/want-to-lose-weight-try-teamwork; "Weight Loss Can Be Contagious, Study Suggests," The Miriam Hospital, February 14, 2012, http://www.miriamhospital.org/wtn/Page.asp?PageID=WTN000161.

Chapter 10: Drafting Your Team

1. Laura Blue, "Obesity Is 'Socially Contagious,' Study Finds," *TIME*, July 25, 2007. http://www.time.com/time/health/article/0,8599,1646997,00.html.

2. Tricia M. Leahey, cited in Brian Dalek, "Your Friends Can Make You Fat," *Men's Health*, June 13, 2011. http://blogs.menshealth.com/health-headlines/friends-and-dieting/2011/06/13.

3. Sirpa Sarlio-Lähteenkorva, Karri Silventoinen and Eero Lahelma, "Relative Weight and Income at Different Levels of Socioeconomic Status," *American Journal of Public Health*, March 2004, vol. 94, no. 3, pp. 468–472.

4. Sue Shellenbarger, "Colleagues Who Can Make You Fat," *The Wall Street Journal*, March 15, 2012. http://online.wsj.com/article/SB10001424052702303717304577279402522090464.html.

5. Ibid.

6. Dr. Rick Kellerman, cited in Miranda Hitti, "Why Men Skip Doctor Visits," WebMD, June 20, 2007. http://men.webmd.com/news/20070620/why-men-skip-doctor-visits.

7. Dr. Allen Dollar, cited in Judy Fortin, "Advice for Men: Don't Wait to See a Doctor," CNN, June 9, 2008. http://edition.cnn.com/2008/HEALTH/06/09/hm.mens.doctors/index.html.

8. Dr. David Dodson, cited in Judy Fortin, "Advice for Men: Don't Wait to See a Doctor."

9. Mike Davison, "Eight Questions Men Are Afraid to Ask Doctors," AskMen.com. http://www.askmen.com/sports/health_60/76c_mens_health.html.

10. Dr. Katherine Krefft, cited in Chris Illades, MD, "Men and Doctors: Understanding the Disconnect," Everyday Health, November 23, 2011. http://www.everydayhealth.com/mens-health/men-and-doctors-understanding-the-disconnect.aspx.

11. Studies conducted in England and Germany showed that vegetarians were about 40 percent less likely to develop cancer compared to meat eaters. In the United States, researchers found significant reductions in cancer risk among those who avoided meat (N. D. Barnard, A. Nicholson and J. L. Howard, "The Medical Costs Attributable to Meat Consumption. Preventative Medicine, 1995, no. 24, pp. 646-655). See "Cancer Prevention and Survival," The Cancer Project. http://www.cancerproject.org/survival/cancer_facts/meat.php.

Chapter 11: Make Your Dash Count

1. R. Sturm, "The Effects of Obesity, Smoking, and Problem Drinking on Chronic Medical Problems and Health Care Costs" *Health Affairs*, 2002, vol. 21, no. 2, pp. 245-253.

2. "Projections of the Population by Selected Age Groups and Sex for the United States: 2010 to 2050," U.S. Census National Population Projections, released 2008 (based on Census 2000). http://www.census.gov/population/www/projections/summarytables.html.

Appendix B: The Top Five Health Numbers to Know

1. Donald Lloyd-Jones, MD, et al., "Heart Disease and Stroke Statistics—2010 Update," The American Heart Association, December 17, 2009. http://circ.ahajournals.org/content/121/ 7/e46. extract.

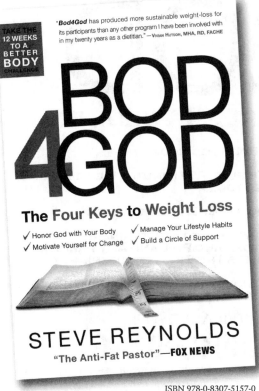

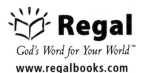

START LIVING...START LOSING

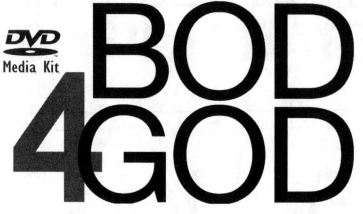

BOD4GOD

DVD Media Kit

FEATURES INCLUDE:

- **COMPLEMENTS THE BOD4GOD BOOK.**

- **FOUR DVD'S WITH TWELVE, 25 - MINUTE VIDEO SESSIONS; PLUS GROUP STARTER TOOLS.**

- **LIFE-CHANGING TALKS FROM STEVE REYNOLDS.**

- **EXPERT INTERVIEWS WITH DOCTORS, TRAINERS, NUTRITIONISTS, PASTORS AND PHIL AND AMY PARHAM (ON SEASON 6 OF NBC'S THE BIGGEST LOSER).**

- **TWELVE BOD4GOD THOUGHTS AND TESTIMONIES. ALSO TWENTY-FOUR BOD4GOD FACTOIDS.**

AVAILABLE AT
WWW.BOD4GOD.ORG
VIDEO PRODUCED BY INNOVATIVE FAITH RESOUCES

FOR MORE INFORMATION
VISIT WWW.BOD4GOD.ORG OR CONTACT

Losing to Live
P.O. Box 300
Merrifield, VA 22116
(703) 635-7100 – (866) 596-6008

You may also contact Pastor Steve Reynolds about speaking to your church or organization.